WHY
MOTHERS'
MEDICATION
MATTERS

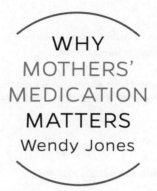

WHY
MOTHERS'
MEDICATION
MATTERS
Wendy Jones

Why Mothers' Medication Matters (Pinter & Martin Why It Matters 8)

First published by Pinter & Martin Ltd 2017

©2017 Wendy Jones

ISBN 978-1-78066-585-6

Also available as ebook

Pinter & Martin Why It Matters ISSN 2056-8657
Series editor: Susan Last
Index: Helen Bilton
Layout: Rebecca Longworth
Cover Design: Blok Graphic, London
Cover Illustration: Donna Smith
Proofreader: Debbie Kennett

British Library Cataloguing-in-Publication Data

A catalogue record for this book is available from the British Library.

Set in Minion

Printed and bound in the UK by Ashford Colour Press Ltd, Gosport, Hampshire

This book has been printed on paper that is sourced and harvested from sustainable forests and is FSC accredited.

Pinter & Martin Ltd
6 Effra Parade
London SW2 1PS
pinterandmartin.com

Contents

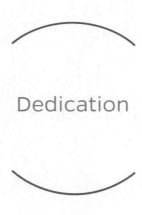

Dedication

This book is dedicated to my wonderful family who support and encourage me every day. Firstly, my wonderful husband of 42 years, Mike, who has supported me emotionally and financially to follow my dreams and my passion for breastfeeding and medication. My incredible daughters Kerensa, Bethany and Tara, who taught me so much about breastfeeding and who have accepted and adopted my passion. My adorable grandchildren Stirling, Isaac and Beatrix, whom I adore with every cell in my body, who have also taken to breastfeeding and taught me even more. My sons-in-law, who haven't just tolerated my idiosyncrasies, but have taken on the passion too and helped me with the IT I needed to write my books and develop my website and Facebook page: Christian, Steve, Rich and Ian, you are the sons I never had. Finally, in remembrance of my mum Peggy, who helped me to begin my breastfeeding journey and encouraged my studies and empowered me to become the person I am, and my dad Dennis, who died far too young but taught me about pharmacy and the value of supporting others.

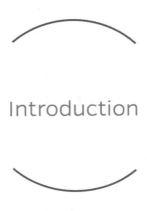

Introduction

The time in a woman's life when she is pregnant, giving birth and breastfeeding is unique, both biologically and emotionally. Women's stories of pregnancy, birth and breastfeeding stay with them for life; they remember how they were treated, how they felt and how they responded to the challenges of motherhood. Even after 30 years as a breastfeeding support worker I am humbled and amazed when women want to tell me their stories. In my work providing evidence-based information about the safety of drugs in breastmilk I hear many women's stories and they inspire me and drive me to continue to support mothers as best I can.

Every day I hear from women who are trying to preserve a breastfeeding relationship with their baby. Some have chronic conditions and need to know how pregnancy and lactation will affect their treatment. Others have experienced sudden illness and want to know whether they can continue to breastfeed while they recover. What they have in common is a desire to do what's right for their baby. It amazes me to see how important breastfeeding is to women: some will even decline necessary treatment for themselves in order to continue. We shouldn't be surprised by this. Breastfeeding *is* important; not just to individual women and babies, but to society as a whole in terms of public health. The evidence that breastfeeding is normal for humans and protects against a host of infections is overwhelming.

However, breastfeeding doesn't come easily to everyone. We may have the equipment, but not everyone has the right support to achieve a pain-free latch. If it hurts we may be told that it doesn't matter, that formula is as good, that a couple of bottles won't hurt to give the nipples a rest and a chance to heal, that dad is willing to feed the baby so mum can get some sleep… and so on. However, much more useful for a mother struggling with breastfeeding is help to find support to make feeding pain-free – from a person who can spend time with the mother and baby, or via internet links, social media or a telephone helpline. Once a baby is well established on the breast and feeding exclusively it is hard to hear that you need to stop, even for a few days; yet this is what many mothers are told when they need medication to treat new or existing health conditions.

A few months ago I was contacted by a mother who had just been diagnosed with cancer and was waiting to start chemotherapy. She had hoped to relactate or pump and dump during her therapy, but had been told that the cancer needed long and aggressive treatment and that this wasn't a realistic plan. She couldn't decide how to go about weaning her baby in the two weeks she had before treatment began: to do so slowly meant having to give her baby bottles of expressed breastmilk or formula when she knew she had milk in her breasts, but to do so rapidly meant she could close her eyes to the diagnosis and pretend for those two weeks that life was normal. She knew she was in denial about the diagnosis. She was aware that if she fed until the last minute she risked having mastitis, or having to express for comfort and throw away the milk just as she started the treatment. Neither option was a good one for her, but in the end she decided that gradual weaning made more sense as she came to terms with her future treatment.

Her story illustrates how breastmilk is more than just a fluid to nourish a baby. It is a magic wand that can calm a toddler who is hurting or anxious. It is a balm to aid sleep. It continues to be a source of antibodies for as long as it continues. Breastfeeding is an intimate relationship between two people that cannot easily be modified. Further, formula milk cannot be compared to breastmilk – from the baby's point of view there are significant disadvantages of a switch to formula made because the mother needs medical treatment, and these should not be overlooked.

If we are to improve the quality of care that mothers receive, we need everyone to understand this. Then, perhaps, it would become less common for mothers to be told to stop breastfeeding when they are ill or need medication.

Sadly, there is a lack of research on the safety of drugs in breastmilk. There are a few specialists who actively collate information on infants exposed to newer drugs via breastmilk. One of these is Tom Hale's Infant Risk Centre in Texas, USA. Generally we rely on very small-scale studies (with at most 20 participants) and even anecdotal reports. To publish a research paper takes time and energy, and these will usually only be undertaken by professionals with a specialist interest in a chronic disease condition. Manufacturers will not usually undertake these studies in line with their lack of requirement to take responsibility for prescription of newer drugs and the ethical dilemma of exposing a third party, who is not unwell, to a drug. With older drugs that have gone out of patent there is no financial benefit to conducting studies when cheaper generic brands of the drug become available. The cost of conducting the trials and producing the data for the MHRA (Medicines and Healthcare products Regulatory Agency) is immense and seen by manufacturers as unjustifiable.

However, does this mean that it is ethically responsible to refuse to treat a mother with medication because she is breastfeeding? I have come across many situations where a mother has been told that if she 'insists' on continuing to breastfeed then she cannot be prescribed adequate pain relief. I was told anecdotally of a maternity hospital ward where mothers were asked on the drug round whether they were breastfeeding or not before analgesics were provided. If they said that they were they were given paracetamol and told that it was all that they could be prescribed. If the mother in the next bed said she was formula-feeding she was told she could have stronger painkillers as she was lucky. What does this do to a mother in pain from episiotomy, stitches, or post-caesarean pain? Is she likely to continue breastfeeding? What messages does it also pass on to her for the future if she becomes ill?

If we are to improve the quality of care that mothers receive, we need everyone to understand the issues that affect pregnant and breastfeeding women. Then, perhaps, it would become less common for mothers to be told to stop breastfeeding when they are ill or need medication.

The remaining sections of this book are a more detailed look at situations affecting mothers who may need medication, using case studies to enable mothers, fathers and grandparents, as well as healthcare professionals, to make informed decisions for each unique mother and baby dyad. My aim is to give women a voice to ask for the help they need to find appropriate treatment without compromising the physical relationship they have with their baby, both in utero and when breastfeeding.

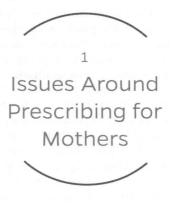

1

Issues Around Prescribing for Mothers

The prescribing of drugs to a pregnant or breastfeeding mother is a potential minefield. Research studies can be difficult to find. The manufacturers of the drugs don't take responsibility for research into the effects on mothers, which means that the person prescribing or selling the drugs has to take professional responsibility for the safety of mother and baby. This is a scary situation for a healthcare professional if they don't know where to look for the evidence, or how to interpret it. This is part of the reason why so many women are told not to take medication in pregnancy, or to breastfeed during treatment. However, it's not the whole story. If a healthcare professional really wants to support a mother, in my experience they will take time to research the safety of the proposed drug and if necessary delay prescribing for a few hours in order to do so. Unfortunately, as my PhD studies showed, personal experience dictates how willing people are to go the extra mile. When offering training to doctors and pharmacists I find the most willing participants are women who have breastfed their own babies. Those with less experience of pregnancy and lactation may be more likely to disregard the issue of prescribing in these circumstances.

Some professionals reassure mothers that *all* drugs are safe and do not mention possible side-effects. This is just as likely to cause concern for a mother. She may become confused when her doctor says one thing, and the pharmacist says another when the prescription is dispensed. The patient information leaflet in the box may say something different too! One GP mother I talked to observed that pharmacists are more risk-averse than doctors, and this may be true. When we sell medicines or dispense prescriptions, most pharmacists stick to strict guidelines. Doctors who have worked in hospitals may have experience with prescribing 'off label' or 'outside of licence' and thus be more comfortable taking these decisions.

One of the difficulties of decision-making on the safety of drugs in breastmilk is that manufacturers cannot undertake clinical trials on the amount of drug which passes into milk. None of us would be willing to expose our babies to medication via our breastmilk when we had no idea of the effect it would have, not only in the short term, but also in the future. The patient information leaflet in virtually every box of tablets, creams, pessaries and inhalers suggests that the drug should not be used by a breastfeeding mother. This is of great concern to mothers – the written word is very powerful and may override information provided by a healthcare professional. When I undertook the research for my PhD in 1995 one mother commented:

> *'I asked the pharmacist in the store if he could suggest a medicine to relieve my diarrhoea. I specifically asked if it was safe for me to take during breastfeeding and he assured me it was. I was really upset when I got home*

to find the leaflet in the box said it shouldn't be used. I trusted him and I was confused.'

The Royal Pharmaceutical Society of Great Britain added a statement to an article I wrote for the *Pharmaceutical Journal* (Jones, 2012) regarding the sale of medication outside of licence (which includes breastfeeding in most cases).

The Royal Pharmaceutical Society reminds pharmacists of principle 1 of the Code of Ethics, which requires them to make the care of the patient their first concern. The Society advises that where a pharmacist is considering making a supply of an OTC medicine outside the terms of its marketing authorisation, the potential risks to the patient of making such a supply and also the potential detriment to the patient of not supplying the medicine must be taken into consideration.

Pharmacists must use their professional judgement as to whether or not to make a supply based on up-to-date clinical guidance, and should always discuss the treatment options with the patient first. If the pharmacist decides to make the supply, he or she must ensure that the patient is counselled appropriately on how to take the medicine because the patient information leaflet may not provide relevant information. The pharmacist should be able to justify his or her actions if called upon to do so.

From this and the discussion above I hope that it is clear that the patient information leaflet is of limited use when we are considering prescribing for pregnant and breastfeeding mothers. If you are concerned, discuss your worries with a pharmacist or doctor, who should be able to access more information.

Healthcare professionals can exert a huge influence on mothers. Many patients rely heavily on what their doctors advise – and rightly so (Saha, 2016). So if a doctor or pharmacist says that it is unsafe to take a drug during pregnancy, or to breastfeed on a drug, mothers are likely to assume that there is a good evidence base on which to base that recommendation. However, prescribing in pregnancy and lactation is a specialist area, and mothers should be aware that the doctors and other healthcare professionals they come into contact with may not have accessed all the information available about the safety of the drug. In this scenario doing your own research, and seeking to communicate openly with your care providers, can be hugely beneficial.

Concerns about the 'purity' of breastmilk

'The doctor told me that the drug would get into my milk. Even though he said it would only be a small amount, I wasn't willing to take it. My baby's health is worth more to me than taking the drugs.'

All of us are anxious to provide the perfect start in life for our babies – it is an innate and natural instinct to protect them. Those of us who choose to breastfeed want to know that our milk is pure and unpolluted, perfect in every way for our baby. How then do we regard taking medication that may get into our milk and pass to our baby?

Some mothers are so scared about what will affect their babies that they not only refuse medication for headaches and colds, preferring to let their bodies heal themselves, but they also question much more simple products. Over the years I have been asked if it is safe to have false nails fitted when breastfeeding, if nail varnish is safe, whether drinking

Ovaltine is safe, and whether a breastfeeding mum can have her hair dyed or straightened.

In pregnancy we bombard women with information on the 'benefits' of breastfeeding. In fact there are no benefits. Consumption of its mother's milk is the biological norm for a mammal. It is in fact artificial formula – prepared from the milk of a different mammal, normally a cow – which is the intervention. As it does not, and cannot, have the biological specificity of breastmilk, it has inherent disadvantages. Formula lacks transport factors such as lactoferrin to facilitate the absorption of iron, oligosaccharides which prevent the attachment of microbes and toxins to the infant gut and urinary tract (the 'protective paint'), the bactericidal and anti-inflammatory activity of lysozyme, the protection of immunoglobulins and many growth factors, to mention just a few of the hundreds of constituents of breastmilk (see Chapter 8). Having made parents aware of these incredible ingredients, which provide the infant with better health outcomes, why do we so readily tell women to stop breastfeeding and introduce formula? Mothers are often told that 'formula is as good as breastmilk these days'. There is no evidence to support this statement. Helen Crawley at First Steps Nutrition Trust has looked at the evidence behind many of the claims made by the formula manufacturers, and shown how flimsy they often are.

When mothers are asked to stop breastfeeding in order to take medication, or worry about a small amount of a drug passing into breastmilk, we need to be mindful of the many constituents of breastmilk that cannot be replicated in infant formula.

Further, breastfeeding is important to mothers and babies. Some healthcare professionals overlook this. Stopping for even a few days may mean that the baby will refuse to go back to the breast, that the mother's milk supply diminishes, that she feels the baby is more settled on the formula (or is told it is by well-meaning others). Breastfeeding is not easily modifiable. It is not a tap to switch off and on again.

When mothers are advised to interrupt or stop breastfeeding unnecessarily there are consequences. Recently I was asked when a mother could return to breastfeeding after a week on flucloxacillin to treat a toenail infection. The nurse who had prescribed had told her she had to stop breastfeeding during the treatment and for five days afterwards. The mother had followed the advice and put her baby onto formula milk. The baby had been sick after most feeds and by day five had developed a rash on her face. When she spoke to a pharmacist they suggested using a different bottle with a very expensive teat to help with the vomiting and a lactose-free milk for the rash. At no time did anyone look into the safety of the standard antibiotic to find out that the mother need never have stopped breastfeeding. When speaking to me the mother burst into tears. She and her baby had been though a week of hell because two healthcare professionals had not looked at the safety of the drug in breastmilk.

In a study in Canada in 1993 a group of 203 mothers was studied (Ito, 1993). They had all been prescribed antibiotics and been reassured by specialist workers that although a small percentage of the drug passed to the baby, it would not be harmful. When 125 of them were followed up 19 of the mothers had chosen not to take the antibiotics and 7 had switched to formula milk while they took the antibiotics, pumping and dumping their milk. Despite having been reassured of the safety of the drug, 1 in 5 women either did not initiate therapy or did not continue breastfeeding. The conclusion of the researchers was that 'Physicians should be aware of the substantial rate of non-compliance with drug regimens among nursing women and the potential negative impact of drug therapy on breastfeeding.'

17

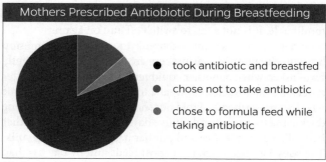

Mothers' actions after being prescribed an antibiotic during pregnancy (Ito, 1993)

Other consequences of interrupting or stopping breastfeeding include:

- What if the baby refuses to drink from a bottle?
- What if you do not have formula available?
- Has anyone provided information on how to maintain your milk supply?
- Do you have a breast pump?
- Is this what you want to do, or would you choose not to take the medication (which may be vitally important for your health)?

The importance of good breastfeeding support alongside medical treatment is clear, and is essential if we want to improve breastfeeding rates and protect the health of mothers and babies in our society.

The dilemma of licensing medication

The manufacturer of any medicinal product must obtain a marketing authorisation from the Licensing Authority prior to promoting and selling the medicine. Part of the application for marketing authorisation includes a clinical expert report, the content of which is governed by European Community legislation (1989). The clinical expert should also discuss 'the possible utilisation during pregnancy and breastfeeding'. A statement on pregnancy and lactation should also appear in the Summary of Product Characteristics. It is not stated what information should be supplied or what, if any, specific animal work is required to generate the data. Animal studies can provide a limited amount of safety data, which may or may not be relevant to human use. In general, little information on the safety of drugs which may pass into a mother's breastmilk is available prior to marketing, so manufacturers will not recommend that a drug should be given to a pregnant or lactating woman. This information is not usually updated, even if subsequent studies present relevant data.

In the USA, the Food and Drug Administration (FDA) is changing labelling to help healthcare professionals assess the risk/benefit of prescription drugs for lactating women (for new drugs from June 2015). The data can come from various sources, including (according to the FDA website) well-conducted studies published in the medical literature about the use of prescription drugs and biological products during pregnancy and breastfeeding. Companies will be required to include clinically relevant information from such studies in the labelling.

The NICE Maternal and Child Nutrition Guideline PH11 (2008) contains a recommendation on prescribing:

- Health professionals and pharmacists who prescribe
  or dispense drugs to a breastfeeding mother should
  consult supplementary sources (for example, the Drugs
  and Lactation Database [LactMed]) or seek guidance
  from the UK Drugs in Lactation Advisory Service.

- Health professionals should discuss the benefits and risks associated with the prescribed medication and encourage the mother to continue breastfeeding, if reasonable to do so. In most cases, it should be possible to identify a suitable medication which is safe to take during breastfeeding by analysing pharmokinetic and study data. The *British National Formulary* should only be used as a guide as it does not contain quantitative data on which to base individual decisions.
- Health professionals should recognise that there may be adverse health consequences for both mother and baby if the mother does not breastfeed. They should also recognise that it may not be easy for the mother to stop breastfeeding abruptly – and that it is difficult to reverse.

This guidance does not seem to have been widely embraced by healthcare professionals. Many continue to consult the *British National Formulary* (BNF), where information on medication often contains the wording 'amount in breastmilk too small to be harmful but manufacturers advise avoid'. Culturally the medical profession is risk averse (as we would want them to be) and very aware of the consequences of adverse events and professional liability. Most healthcare professionals have very little training in breastfeeding, let alone the safety of drugs in breastmilk or during pregnancy. Many are not aware of the databases and reference sources available in this specialist area.

Over the past 20 years of running the Drugs in Breastmilk service, I have provided evidence-based information for healthcare professionals and parents, sometimes interpreted in light of my experience. If the FDA's approach to labelling were to be implemented elsewhere, life might become less challenging for mothers trying to stay well and protect their babies. As parents we need to have full information on the amount of drug that passes into milk, outcomes in babies exposed to it and any adverse effects, for example loose bowel motions after antibiotics, including any which need to be reported to a medical professional. In the latter case Yellow Cards should be submitted to the MHRA so that knowledge is updated. These can be submitted by mothers, as well as healthcare professionals, for prescribed drugs, over-the-counter drugs and herbal remedies.

Training for healthcare professionals

The Unicef UK Baby Friendly Initiative developed a GP training package which was made available in some areas. The aim was to equip GPs with:

- A basic understanding of how breastfeeding works
- Knowledge of how to treat common breast conditions (mastitis, thrush, etc.)
- Knowledge of how to access a reliable reference source for prescribing drugs for breastfeeding mothers

I wrote a similar training pack for the Breastfeeding Network. A research project was undertaken by a medical student in 2012 to evaluate the impact of the training. (Aubrey-Jones, 2012).

One hundred and forty-eight GP practices in Hampshire and 58 practices within Berkshire West were sent links to the pack. Those who completed a pre- and post-training questionnaire showed an increase in knowledge of 10%. In addition 75% said they would recommend the package to others. However, the number who completed the pre- and post-training questionnaire was dismally low: 15 completed and returned the pre-training questionnaire, with just 7 going on to complete and return the post training questionnaire. Twenty-four completed a Survey Monkey form about any breastfeeding education they had received and their attitudes towards future breastfeeding education. Thirty-six percent of respondents said they had had 'hardly any' or 'no' previous breastfeeding education. However, only 27% of respondents said they would definitely consider further education.

Some of the findings were particularly interesting:

- When asked about the benefits of breastfeeding, 90% knew that breastfed babies have a lower risk of obesity later in life and 86% were aware that breastfeeding provides long-term benefits to a mother's health. However, 14% of GPs did not know that artificially fed babies are more susceptible to gastroenteritis, as compared to breastfed babies. The majority (81%) knew that the risk of breast and ovarian cancer is lower among women who have breastfed.
- 63% of GPs were unable to recognise that one-sided breast pain is not a symptom of thrush.
- When asked about sore nipples, 41% of GPs incorrectly thought that sore nipples could be an inevitable part of breastfeeding.
- When asked about treatment of mastitis, 19% of GPs incorrectly thought that antibiotics are always indicated. More encouragingly, almost all of GPs (97%) knew that mothers with mastitis should be advised to continue breastfeeding.
- 37% of GPs weren't sure of the safety of ibuprofen in breastfeeding. This is particularly concerning given that 92% of GPs had just reported that they felt confident prescribing for breastfeeding mothers. Of the GPs who didn't know about the safety of ibuprofen in breastfeeding, all had reported that they were confident prescribing for breastfeeding mothers.

All those who completed the e-learning had had children and 87% of them said their children had been breastfed. The majority of those who undertook the learning (75%) were female.

A 2011 paper by Hussain reported:

> 'The decision-making process between health professionals and women is usually not a negotiated process, and women are often asked to stop breastfeeding whilst taking a medicine. Women, in turn, are left dissatisfied with the advice received, many choosing not to initiate therapy or not to continue breastfeeding.'

This highlights some of the problems we currently face when advocating for care for women that takes account of their breastfeeding status. Better education for GPs, and clearer pathways of referral to skilled breastfeeding support, could improve the situation immensely. This is essential when breastfeeding rates are being used as a marker of public health in the UK.

Media reporting on the safety of medication

Reports in the media also have an impact on the use of medication in pregnancy and during breastfeeding. Einarson et al (2005) examined the impact of an advisory notice issued by Health Canada on the potential adverse effects on newborns of their mothers taking SSRI antidepressants in pregnancy. The media had reported the story, and we all know that newspapers and websites prefer sensationalist headlines to simple facts. Mothers who called the Motherisk Programme in Toronto seeking information on the safety of SSRI antidepressants during the study period were asked to complete a questionnaire. The study followed up 43 of 49 women (88%) who contacted the programme. All callers reported that the media coverage had caused anxiety. Seven misunderstood the information (their children were more than a year old); five had discontinued their antidepressant (three stopped abruptly, although two later restarted after speaking to counsellors, and two with some form of tapering off), while six were considering stopping but decided to continue following reassurance from the team. The researchers commented that *'They all felt that this was important information to know, however would not have been so alarmed if it had been translated by the media in a less "scary" fashion'*. I urge everyone to exercise caution when reports appear in the media; it is always worth looking more closely at the source research papers and seeking advice if you are worried.

Pregnancy and breastfeeding for mothers with pre-existing medical conditions

In today's society women can contemplate pregnancy despite pre-existing medical conditions if their symptoms are well controlled by medication. This may include mothers who have heart conditions, have had transplants, or have cystic fibrosis or multiple sclerosis. Every woman deserves to be supported through pregnancy and enabled to breastfeed if she chooses. Women with existing conditions may need pre-conception counselling to take additional folic acid, or to change or stop their medication in light of the available (or not!) safety data. For example, sodium valproate in epilepsy is implicated in birth abnormalities and so should not be used by pregnant women unless it is absolutely unavoidable.

I am continually unpleasantly surprised to be contacted by pregnant women who are nearing their due date but have never been given the opportunity to discuss evidence-based information on the safety of the drug(s) they are taking if they choose to breastfeed. I have been called by midwives who tell me that they have a mum in labour but that no one knows if she can breastfeed after the birth. She has been pregnant for nine months! Why is there not a care plan in place?

If a mother has a condition such as diabetes, in which milk production (lactogenesis II) may be delayed, has she been shown how to hand express her colostrum from week 36 and freeze it ready for use postnatally if necessary? Is she aware that she may need to consume more carbohydrate when she is breastfeeding, and that night snacks should be readily available even in the maternity unit? When I was conducting my research (Jones, 2000) I met an insulin-dependent mother who had experienced a hypoglycaemic episode the night after she gave birth. She had decided to stop breastfeeding her baby in case her breastmilk was 'inadequate' if her glycaemic control was unstable. When we talked I discovered that she had not eaten since 6pm the previous evening and no foods were available to her overnight on the postnatal ward, so her blood glucose sugars had plummeted. She had not thought to take food with her for her postnatal stay. While this was more than 15 years ago, and I hope that such a situation would no longer occur in our hospitals, it illustrates the problems that can arise if the needs of a mother with a chronic medical condition are not carefully considered.

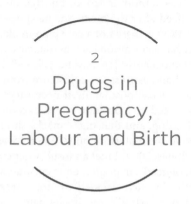

2

Drugs in Pregnancy, Labour and Birth

There are many situations that occur today that did not exist when I began my studies. As more women breastfeed, and for longer, the number of complex (from the point of view of medication) situations they can encounter has increased. Mothers wanting to get pregnant while breastfeeding may seek fertility treatment, and mothers breastfeeding longer term may develop conditions that require medication. In this chapter I explore some of these situations and show how 'mother-friendly' solutions can be found if those involved in a woman's care are able to access good information and apply it sensitively.

Breastfeeding and assisted conception

Many families now seek help to conceive, using a variety of drugs and procedures. With these much-wanted babies, it is perhaps not surprising that when planning a second pregnancy mothers are in no hurry to wean their first baby from the breast. For most women frequent breastfeeding suppresses ovulation and the return of periods, which many see as an advantage.

But for those in a hurry to become pregnant, or who know that they may need assistance to conceive, it is important that they begin to ovulate. Some mothers try to drop feeds in order to stimulate a return to a normal menstrual cycle, or use herbal remedies or drugs to bring on periods.

A wide variety of drugs are used to assist conception, many of which have not been studied in breastfeeding. Thus we have to look at the theoretical levels in breastmilk and the absorption from the gastro-intestinal tract rather than evidence from studies. Many cycles of IVF involve high-dose oestrogen, and the risk from these is a reduction in the mother's milk supply. This may sound undesirable, but bear in mind that a woman's milk supply is likely to drop if she becomes pregnant, so in this case the medication may just bring forward a situation that might soon occur anyway.

Many clinics ask that mothers have stopped breastfeeding for two months before they embark on IVF treatment. This is said to be because of the need to give the new pregnancy the best possible chance of implanting and developing, but the evidence behind the recommendation seems weak. Mothers can naturally become pregnant again while still breastfeeding. Breastfeeding itself does not harm a pregnancy unless it is already so vulnerable that it is unlikely to continue anyway. It has often been suggested that the release of oxytocin during the let-down of milk could contribute to uterine contractions and expulsion of the foetus, but we know that lots of things, for example orgasm, result in the release of oxytocin, and women are not advised to avoid these.

There is a very active Facebook group where mothers who are still breastfeeding and are undergoing assisted conception support each other. Peer support is a powerful tool. I lurk in the background of this group providing support when requested (www.facebook.com/groups/bfduringivf/)

Breastfeeding a toddler when you are pregnant

It should come as no surprise to health professionals that women who become pregnant may be breastfeeding a toddler. The World Health Organization's infant feeding recommendation (2002) says:

> *'Breastfeeding is an unequalled way of providing ideal food for the healthy growth and development of infants; it is also an integral part of the reproductive process with important implications for the health of mothers. As a global public health recommendation, infants should be exclusively breastfed for the first six months of life to achieve optimal growth, development and health.*
>
> *Thereafter, to meet their evolving nutritional requirements, infants should receive nutritionally adequate and safe complementary foods while breastfeeding continues for up to two years of age or beyond.'*

We know that the early stages of pregnancy bring nausea and even hyperemesis for up to 70% of women (Lee, 2000). Symptoms can occur at any time of the day and dealing with an active toddler at home or, worse, trying to work and look after a toddler, does not allow for slow morning starts nibbling on ginger biscuits. The email below is typical of enquiries I receive on the subject:

> *'I am 7 weeks pregnant and suffering from nausea. My toddler is still heavily reliant on breastfeeding even though she is 18 months old. My GP told me that she doesn't need breastmilk any longer and that it has no goodness in it but I am sure this is not true. She loves her booby and is just not ready to stop yet and to be honest neither am I. It is the only way I can settle her when I feel so sick. Is there any drug I can take and carry on*

breastfeeding? My doctor said not but I don't think he is very supportive of me breastfeeding at this stage.'

Firstly, we know that breastfeeding an 18-month-old is beneficial for both mother and child. Secondly, when mothers are given wrong information about breastfeeding, they begin to doubt the advice they are given about medication, which is of concern because we all need to have confidence in the person responsible for our own and our children's health. Mothers in this situation seek other sources of support. Many of them find their way to me via email or Facebook, but many others end up googling or asking advice from others. The internet is a wonderful source of information, but it is hard to know what is 'good information'. Nausea in pregnancy resolves by 16 weeks in 90% of cases. Hyperemesis gravidarum occurs in less than 1% of pregnancies, but often involves the mother being admitted for rehydration and symptom control with medication, as the Duchess of Cambridge discovered in her first pregnancy.

In my experience, GPs are often happy to prescribe anti-emetics, but only if the mother weans her nursling, which she is often reluctant to do abruptly. The saddest messages I get are from mothers who have been told that they have to stop breastfeeding in order to be prescribed any anti-sickness medication, but when challenged the doctors admit that they don't know and are erring on the side of caution. When a drug is safe enough for a six-week-old foetus to be exposed to, is it justifiable to worry about the exposure a two-and-a-half year-old toddler, breastfeeding maybe just to sleep, will get through breastmilk? Better education would improve the care mothers get in this scenario. For mothers who have become pregnant, suffer from nausea and are still breastfeeding the support group Pregnancy Sickness Support is useful (www.pregnancysicknesssupport.org.uk).

Some drugs used to treat nausea

Cyclizine is a type of antihistamine that can make a toddler drowsy and theoretically eventually reduce the milk supply due to reduced length of feeding time. It is often the first drug tried for nausea in pregnancy.

Promethazine is also an antihistamine and can elicit pronounced drowsiness with a risk of making a toddler drowsy and theoretical lowering of supply (as above). No increased risks of congenital abnormalities in the baby above the background rate for the population have been reported when cyclizine or promethazine have been used in therapeutic doses (NICE CKS 2013).

Prochlorperazine levels in breastmilk have not been measured, but members of this family of drugs penetrate breastmilk in low levels. No increased risks of congenital abnormalities, above the background rate for the population, have been reported when prochlorperazine has been used in therapeutic doses (NICE CKS 2013).

Metoclopramide reaches breastmilk in low levels and has also been used in the past to increase low milk supply. It is not recommended in mothers younger than 20, as they are more likely to experience side-effects. No side-effects have been noted in babies exposed to metoclopramide though breastmilk and it is widely given directly to children. No increased risks of congenital abnormalities, above the background rate for the population, have been reported when metoclopramide has been used in therapeutic doses (NICE CKS 2013), although one cohort study has shown a higher incidence of premature delivery after metoclopramide exposure.

Domperidone passes into breastmilk in low levels and is used to increase milk supply. However, some concerns have been raised by the Medicines and Healthcare products Regulatory Agency on its safety and the risk of producing abnormal heart rhythms. Some doctors may feel less comfortable prescribing it, but the amount passing into breastmilk will not harm your nursling.

Pyridoxine (vitamin B6) when compared with placebo may be effective at reducing nausea, but not vomiting. However, the evidence is of low quality (Mazzotta, 2000). Although no relationship has been found between B6 status and the incidence of morning sickness, using 10–40mg/day appears to reduce the severity of symptoms and is often used as a benchmark to evaluate other treatments. Doses of over 200mg a day are discouraged as sensory neuropathy (loss of sensation in the fingers) is reported with high doses given for extended periods.

Ondansetron has not been studied in breastmilk. However, this drug is widely used to treat severe vomiting in children undergoing chemotherapy. Levels of any drugs reaching breastmilk are smaller than licensed paediatric doses. Observe the breastfed baby for sedation, irritability, diarrhoea or constipation and urinary retention. Most studies have found no increased risks of congenital abnormalities above the background rate for the population when ondansetron is used in therapeutic doses. However, a single study has shown an increased risk of isolated cleft palate following first-trimester exposure to ondansetron, which is why it is usually the drug used when all else has failed and the mother and baby are at risk from dehydration.

For more information please see the information available in Ebrahimi, 2010.

Many mothers who become pregnant while breastfeeding are, in my experience, subjected to diatribes about the lack of benefit of breastmilk for toddlers, the risk to the pregnancy of continued breastfeeding, and utter disbelief that anyone breastfeeds a baby longer than six months, let alone for a year and beyond. This is unacceptable and I hope that all those working to advocate for breastfeeding succeed in their aim to improve our cultural and medical understanding of breastfeeding. Our health professionals need to know that breastfeeding to two and beyond is normal and advantageous for mother and baby. Also, once a mother becomes pregnant again her breastmilk supply usually starts to dwindle and may cease until colostrum begins to be produced for the new baby. It is common for breastfeeding to become painful as nipples become sensitive, and some mother and toddler pairs stop breastfeeding at this point. Other dyads continue to enjoy breastfeeding throughout the pregnancy and go on to tandem feed. The breasts revert to producing colostrum and just the right milk for the new baby, which is fine for the toddler too. The milk usually comes in much faster because of the dual stimulation. Most families find that the toddler is happy to let the baby feed first, or both children feed together, one at each breast. There are no rules; it depends on what works for the family.

Drugs in labour

A variety of drugs may be offered to a mother in labour, depending on whether she is being induced, is in natural labour, is progressing well or is struggling.

Normal labour

In a normal labour that has begun naturally and is progressing well, there is no reason why a breastfeeding mother may not continue to feed her older baby if she so desires. It will release some oxytocin, which may help. This is similar to suggestions that nipple stimulation may accelerate labour. I'm not sure that there is a massive research evidence base behind this, but if it feels right then it is OK! During a natural labour a mother may not need any medication. In hospital she may be offered an opiate tablet like dihydrocodeine or rely on gas and air. Other options are discussed below. However, not all labours progress 'naturally'.

Induction of labour

There are many reasons for induction of labour: being 'overdue', or concerns over the health of mum or baby (particularly high blood pressure, spontaneous rupture of membranes without labour beginning, diabetes, growth of the baby slowing). Most women go into labour spontaneously by 42 weeks (NICE 2008).

Many inductions beyond 40 weeks of pregnancy begin with a sweep of the cervix by the midwife to encourage it to thin and open. Pharmacologically most inductions commence with vaginal application of a prostaglandin gel or tablet or controlled-release pessary (the latter is intended to act over a period of 24 hours). If labour has not begun within six hours then a further dose may be given. Prostaglandins are drugs that help to induce labour by encouraging the cervix to soften and shorten (ripen). This allows the cervix to open and contractions to start. The drugs used to induce labour should not affect your subsequent breastfeeding.

Augmenting labour

If further help is still needed to augment labour you may be given synthetic oxytocin (Syntocinon) via a drip. The rate at which the drug is given can be adjusted according to your response. However, the use of oxytocin speeds up the intensity of contractions quite rapidly compared to natural labour and you may find your need for pain relief is greater. A recent study (Brimdyr, 2015) has shown that use of synthetic oxytocin significantly decreased the likelihood of the baby suckling while in skin-to-skin during the first hour after birth. That does not, however, mean that you should be unduly worried if your labour needs to be augmented. It could well be that the rapid and more painful nature of augmented labours affected how the mothers felt after delivery. Unrestricted skin-to-skin is the best way to stimulate good milk supply and assist your baby in latching. Even if you don't manage a good breastfeed in the first hour, it doesn't mean that it won't happen later, and you can access breastfeeding support to help you.

Pain relief for a caesarean section

Many caesareans now take place as epidural deliveries using fentanyl, although in an emergency an operation under general anaesthetic may be necessary. The drugs used in general anaesthetics pass out of the body in a very short space of time and, if the health of mother and baby permits, the baby may be put to the mother's breast while she is still in recovery. More and more frequently babies are placed in skin-to-skin in the operating theatre, allowing the breast crawl and first feed to take place just as in a natural birth.

In theatre most women are given an injection or a suppository of morphine to provide pain relief over a number of hours after surgery. Others may be given diclofenac as a suppository. Post-operatively analgesia depends on the mother's needs, but may include Oramorph liquid, patient-controlled morphine, regular paracetamol plus a non-steroidal drug (naproxen, diclofenac or ibuprofen), tramadol or dihydrocodeine. All of these can be taken by a breastfeeding mother although the reaction of the baby to any opiate drugs (e.g. morphine) should be monitored. If the baby becomes excessively sleepy or reluctant to feed, the painkillers should be reconsidered.

It can be very difficult to move around after a caesarean, including lifting the baby to feed, so the importance of pain relief should not be underestimated. If you take opiate painkillers you may also suffer from constipation; keep your fluid levels up and eat fruit and vegetables. If you need laxatives to help, those that help to bulk and soften should be used sooner rather than later. You can take these and breastfeed as normal.

Painkillers in labour

Some women feel the need for pain relief in labour – that might be paracetamol or something stronger. You may be offered dihdyrocodeine tablets or an injection of pethidine or diamorphine.

Pethidine is less frequently used now than it was 40 years ago. The timing of the administration of pethidine is important. If it is given within three hours of birth, the baby may be born affected by the amount transferred through the placenta. Hogg et al estimated in 1977 that if given late in labour the baby may continue to be affected for two to three days, because the newborn's liver and kidneys are too immature to metabolise it effectively. While the half-life of pethidine in an adult is less than four hours, in a newborn it has a median half-life of 11 hours, but studies have measured times up to 60 hours. The baby may be very drowsy after delivery and reluctant to feed, risking hypoglycaemia as well as missing multiple opportunities to stimulate the mother's milk supply. In a report by the National Birthday Trust (Chamberlain, 1993), 36.9% received pethidine in labour. Rajan (1994) concluded that apart from general anaesthetics it is 'the most inhibiting drug to breastfeeding', causing drowsiness in the mother and baby.

Alternatives include injections of diamorphine, which

has a much shorter half-life than pethidine. It is converted to 6-acetylmorphine and thence to morphine. As with all opiates there are risks of sedation and respiratory depression in the baby. I have been asked several times about the effect of diamorphine on breastfeeding, but have found few studies apart from those looking at drug-misusing mothers. As an analgesic, morphine is generally considered to be an ideal choice for breastfeeding mothers when used post-operatively or for other forms of pain 'in normal dosage ranges'. Diamorphine is much less frequently used than pethidine.

The Chamberlain study also reported on Apgar scores following the use of drugs in labour.

Drugs used in labour	Apgar score less than 7 at 1 minute	Apgar score less than 7 at 5 minutes
Diamorphine	12.30%	2.30%
Pethidine	12.30%	1.30%
Entonox	9.10%	1.20%
No drug	7.50%	1.00%

Apgar scores following use of drugs in labour (Chamberlain, 1993)

Epidural

This involves the injection of an anaesthetic into the epidural space in the spine via a very fine needle. The anaesthetic numbs the spinal nerves, blocking the pain signals from the lower part of the body. Epidurals are widely used in caesarean sections to allow the mother to be aware of the birth of her baby. They normally contain fentanyl or sometimes remifentanil. Epidurals can cause your blood pressure to drop, making you feel dizzy and sick. Some studies have found that epidurals cause babies to feed less frequently after delivery. One study (Beilin, 2005) has shown that doses of fentanyl over 150 microgrammes resulted in lower breastfeeding rates at six weeks.

Meptid (meptazinol) is claimed to cause less sedation than pethidine. It is significantly more expensive and appears to be offered less frequently. In one double-blind study of the two drugs (Sheikh, 1986) in 205 women there was no difference between the two drugs with respect to pain relief or side-effects in mother or baby. In a randomised double-blind study of 1,100 women (Morrison, 1987) there was no difference in the analgesia provided by the two drugs; the pattern of side-effects was similar, but the incidence of vomiting was greater following meptazinol administration. The babies in the two groups were similar with respect to resuscitation received, weight gains or losses and the incidence of clinical neonatal jaundice. The most striking findings were the poor quality of pain relief experienced by both groups following parenteral analgesics and the high incidence of side-effects.

No two labours are the same. Follow your instincts, but remember that often when you think you can't cope without pain relief any more, the birth is imminent. Make sure you and your partner have discussed pain relief beforehand and that he reminds you if you were very determined not to have any.

If your baby is drowsy after delivery and slow to feed, make sure that you stimulate your milk supply with hand expression and drop the colostrum into the baby's mouth with a syringe or teaspoon. This keeps the baby's sugar levels up and will help him or her to wake up and feed directly. Also keep the baby in skin-to-skin and use every flicker of an eyelid as a cue to offer the breast.

Non-pharmacological options for pain relief in labour

Gas and air (Entonox) is widely used (approximately 80% of mothers) in well-established labour. It provides some detachment from the pain. It is composed of half nitrous oxide (laughing gas) and half oxygen. It does not affect your unborn baby. It is impossible to overuse it. If you breathe in too much you become drowsy and let the mouthpiece go.

TENS machines provide small pulses of electric current through pads placed on your skin. It is postulated that the pulses block pain signals from reaching the brain or stimulate the release of endorphins. There is a lack of good research on the benefits of TENS machines, but some women find them very helpful.

Managed delivery of the placenta

Syntocinon (oxytocin) can be given to manage the third stage of labour. The injection is given just after the birth of the baby to stimulate the womb to contract. This helps the placenta to separate from the womb, speeds up delivery of the placenta and reduces the risk of heavy bleeding. Syntocinon may pass into breastmilk in small amounts, but as oxytocin is a normal component of breastmilk and one of the hormones needed to produce it, there will be no harmful effect on the newborn baby. It is rapidly inactivated in the baby's gut.

Drugs used following post-partum haemorrhage

Postpartum bleeding or postpartum haemorrhage (PPH) is often defined as the loss of more than 500ml or 1,000ml of blood within the first 24 hours following childbirth. It is sometimes recommended that babies of mothers who have received syntometrine (ergometrine and oxytocin) do not receive breastmilk for 12 hours, and that the mother should pump and dump her colostrum, on the grounds that ergometrine is secreted into milk and the inhibitory effect of ergometrine on prolactin can cause a reduction in milk secretion. There are no reports of adverse events from babies exposed to syntometrine and no justification for interrupting breastfeeding. Methylergonovine is more widely used in the USA. The LactMed website says:

> 'Limited information indicates that maternal doses of methylergonovine up to 0.75mg daily produce low levels in milk. Product labelling in the US currently recommends avoiding breastfeeding for 12 hours following the last dose of methylergonovine. This warning appears to be based on unpublished adverse reactions in breastfed infants after several days of maternal methylergonovine therapy. The use of shorter courses of the drug after delivery during the colostral phase of lactation would not be expected to transfer appreciable amounts of drug to the breastfed infant or risk adverse effects in the infant.'

Extreme loss of blood (life-threatening bleeding requiring blood transfusion) may lead to Sheehan's syndrome. This may lead to very low milk production and low blood pressure, as well as fatigue. It is rare but should be investigated if there has been a large blood loss at delivery and the mother is struggling to breastfeed.

Anti-hypertensives in pregnancy and breastfeeding

Raised blood pressure in pregnancy is often a sign of pre-eclampsia. It reduces the blood flow through the placenta to the baby and can result in intra-uterine growth retardation (IUGR) so that the baby may be born small for dates. It is important to be aware that headaches and visual disturbances may reflect a worsening of the condition and require urgent medical attention, which may involve delivery of the baby at

37–38 weeks of pregnancy.

The most commonly used anti-hypertensive drug is labetolol. This is a beta-blocker that passes into breastmilk at low levels and can be continued after delivery. Beta-blockers are associated with changes in blood sugar levels and it is usual to monitor babies exposed to these drugs carefully after delivery. This may involve measurement of blood sugar levels, but should include encouraging regular breastfeeds (or hand expression of colostrum to stimulate a good milk supply) and assessment of attachment by someone with expertise in breastfeeding. Such monitoring is not related simply to the drug, but also to the fact that the baby may be low weight and delivered early.

Other drugs used to reduce blood pressure include nifedipine and methyldopa, both of which pass into breastmilk in low levels and should not affect the baby.

Antibiotics post-delivery

Because caesarean sections involve a surgical incision, a single injection of antibiotics will normally be given in theatre to minimise the risk of infection. These will be suitable for breastfeeding and should not affect your baby.

Antibiotics may also be prescribed for wound infections or delay in healing of episiotomy. They may also be suggested for mastitis (see pages 91–94).

Homeopathic remedies

Homeopathic Arnica is taken by some mothers to reduce bruising and aid healing following delivery. The amount passing through breastmilk is minuscule and will not affect the baby.

Deep-vein thrombosis

The risk of developing a clot in your legs persists for six weeks after birth, which is why in some women with a combination of risk factors, such as caesarean and excess weight (BMI over 30), multiple birth, or being a smoker, there may be routine prescription of injections to thin the blood. These are usually called low molecular weight heparins and include dalteparin (Fragmin), enoxaparin (Clexane), and tinzaparin (Innohep). These all have large molecules and are poorly absorbed from the gut, so do not affect your ability to breastfeed as normal.

The symptoms of a clot in your leg (usually only one) are:

- Swelling
- Pain
- Warm skin
- Tenderness
- Redness, particularly at the back of the leg below the knee

Occasionally after birth you may feel breathless, or have a cough and chest pain. On examination you may have low oxygen saturation measurements, which suggest that a clot has been formed or moved to the lungs. You may need an X-ray, CT scan with contrast (no risk with breastfeeding) or a ventilation perfusion scan.

A pulmonary ventilation perfusion scan is actually two tests that are usually performed together. These use inhaled and injected radioactive material to measure breathing and circulation in all areas of the lungs. There is a small exposure to radiation from the radioisotope used in this scan. The risk to you is about the same as having an X-ray. The radioisotopes are short-lived and leave the body quickly.

In the first test, radioactive material is breathed in and pictures or images are taken to look at the airflow in the lungs. In the second part, a different radioactive material is injected into a vein in the arm, and more images are taken to see the blood flow in the lungs. The standard advice is to stop breastfeeding for 24 hours, but these pieces of information are available from expert sources.

Diagnostic Procedure:	Lung ventilation Imaging
Radiopharmaceuticals:	99m TC-DPAA (labelled aerosol)
T½ hours:	6 hours
Dosage Range:	30 MSV
Breastfeeding restrictions to limit exposure to <1 MSV*:	No interruption for 30 MCI or less[1]
Breastfeeding restrictions to limit exposure to zero MSV*	30 hours

*a millisievert (MSV) is defined as 'the average accumulated background radiation dose to an individual for a year'

Recommended time to interrupt breastfeeding after lung perfusion (Hale, Medications and Mothers Milk 2014 Appendix).

Test:	Lung perfusion
Radiopharmaceutical:	99mTcA-MAA
Advice to patient:	13 hour interruption to feeding

Recommended time to interrupt breastfeeding after lung ventilation imaging. Taken from www.insideradiology.com.au

LactMed states:

'*Summary of Use during Lactation Technetium MAA: Information in this record refers to the use of technetium Tc 99m albumin aggregated (Tc 99m macro aggregated albumin; Tc 99m MAA) as a diagnostic agent. Breastfeeding should be interrupted for 12 to 12.6 hours after administration of Tc 99m albumin aggregated. During the period of interruption, the breasts should be emptied regularly and completely. If the mother has expressed and saved milk prior to the examination, she can feed it to the infant during the period of nursing interruption. The milk that is pumped by the mother during the time of breastfeeding interruption can either be discarded or stored refrigerated and given to the infant after 10 physical half-lives, or about 60 hours, have elapsed.*'

Another LactMed entry states:

'*Technetium DTPA: Information in this record refers to the use of technetium Tc 99m pentetate (Tc 99m-diethylenetriaminepentaacetic acid; Tc 99m DTPA) as a diagnostic agent. The United States Nuclear Regulatory Commission states that breastfeeding need not be interrupted after administration of Tc 99m DTPA in doses up to 1000 MBq (30 mCi) intravenously or by inhalation to a nursing mother. The International Commission on Radiological Protection also recommends that breastfeeding need not be interrupted after administration of technetium Tc 99m pentetate. However, to follow the principle of keeping exposure 'as low as reasonably achievable', some experts recommend nursing the infant just before administration of the radiopharmaceutical and interrupting breastfeeding for three to six hours after the dose, then expressing the milk completely once and discarding it. If the mother has expressed and saved milk prior to the examination, she can feed it to the infant during the period of nursing interruption. Mothers need not refrain from close contact with their infants after usual clinical doses.'*

99mTc-diethylenetriaminepentaacetic acid (DTPA) is the most commonly used radiopharmaceutical in the aerosol, while the radiopharmaceutical used for perfusion imaging is 99mTc-MAA (Parker, 2012).

So one local guideline recommends seven hours, two others recommend 12 hours and the Royal Australian and New Zealand College of Radiologists recommends 24 hours! Confused? I am too, but what is clear is that 24 hours is not supported by the research evidence and information from experts on radioactivity. I have included the references above so you can discuss with your clinicians.

Stillbirth and milk production

At some births sadly there is no baby to take home; some babies are born sleeping or die soon after birth. In this situation the mother's body will initiate milk production as normal. In the past medical professionals often prescribed drugs like bromocriptine and cabergoline to dry up the milk as quickly as possible. These drugs have very severe side-effects, including vomiting, postural hypotension, fatigue, dizziness and dry mouth. Also, particularly with high doses, women may suffer confusion, psychomotor excitation, hallucinations; rarely diarrhoea, gastro-intestinal bleeding, gastric ulcer, abdominal pain, tachycardia, bradycardia, arrhythmia, insomnia, psychosis, visual disturbances, and tinnitus. Cabergoline can also cause depression. They should be avoided if the mother has experienced pre-eclampsia. Both drugs can produce sudden onset sleep or excessive daytime drowsiness, and driving should be avoided.

The *BNF* contains a warning on the use of bromocriptine:

> *Postpartum or puerperium*
> *Should not be used postpartum or in puerperium in women with high blood pressure, coronary artery disease, or symptoms (or history) of serious mental disorder; monitor blood pressure carefully (especially during first few days) in postpartum women. Very rarely hypertension, myocardial infarction, seizures or stroke (both sometimes preceded by severe headache or visual disturbances), and mental disorders have been reported in postpartum women given bromocriptine for lactation suppression – caution with antihypertensive therapy and avoid other ergot alkaloids. Discontinue immediately if hypertension, unremitting headache, or signs of CNS toxicity develop.*

Although bromocriptine and cabergoline are licensed to suppress lactation, they are not recommended for routine suppression when women have decided not to breastfeed, or for the relief of symptoms of postpartum pain and engorgement that can be adequately treated with simple analgesics and breast support. If a dopamine-receptor agonist is required, cabergoline is preferred.

The FDA-approved indication for the use of bromocriptine for lactation suppression has been withdrawn, and it is no longer approved for this purpose due to numerous maternal deaths. In 2015, the French pharmacovigilance programme published a review of the adverse events associated with bromocriptine use to cease lactation. This group reported 105 serious adverse reactions including cardiovascular (70.5%), neurological (14.4%) and psychiatric (8.6%) events. There were also two fatalities: one 32-year-old female had a myocardial infarction with an arrhythmia, and a 21-year-old female had an ischaemic stroke (reported in Hale online, accessed August 2016).

Ectopic pregnancies

An ectopic pregnancy is when a fertilised egg implants itself outside the womb, usually in one of the fallopian tubes. The pregnancy is not viable and the mother's health is at risk if it continues. Sadly the pregnancy has to be removed, either surgically, often as an emergency, or by using medication (normally methotrexate). If the mother is still breastfeeding an older baby this has to be interrupted for 24 hours after taking the drug. This can be very difficult for a mother emotionally, having lost an early pregnancy and having to manage a toddler who cannot understand why milk is not available. A lack of sympathy from a health professional who does not understand why you would want to breastfeed a toddler can make this type of situation even worse.

I was recently contacted by a mother who wanted information on how to sustain her lactation. She had experienced an ectopic pregnancy and been told that she could not breastfeed her six-and-a-half-month old baby for *three months*. She was determined that this was not to be the end of their breastfeeding relationship and had decided to pump and dump for three months and then to go back to breastfeeding her baby, who would then be 10 months old. She was delighted to learn she could return to breastfeeding immediately, but very angry that her breastfeeding experience could have been destroyed by being given incorrect, non-evidence-based information.

Breastfeeding and the morning-after pill

It is all too easy to forget about the risk of getting pregnant when you have an older baby and little opportunity to relax and spend time with your partner. When reality bites and you realise that you have had unprotected sex it is helpful to know that you can take the morning-after pill levonorgestrel (Levonelle) and continue to breastfeed as normal. There is no information on the amount of the newer drug ulipristal (ellaOne) passing into breastmilk, although data from the manufacturer indicates that the amounts in breastmilk are low. World Health Organization guidelines state that women who are breastfeeding can generally use ulipristal as an emergency contraceptive. The manufacturer reports that after this medication was given to 12 breastfeeding women for emergency contraception the mean concentration of ulipristal and its metabolite in milk were 22.7ng/mL and 4.49ng/mL in the first 24 hours. Using this data on the mean ulipristal concentration in the first 24 hours of therapy, the relative infant dose was 0.8%, well below the 10% level considered safe (Hale). Your next period may be early or late, and barrier contraception should be continued until the next period. Levonorgestrel can be purchased over the counter from a pharmacist or prescribed by a GP, family planning clinic or accident and emergency department. Should your next period be delayed by more than five days you should seek further medical advice. Levonelle is reported by the manufacturers not to show evidence of teratogenicity (harm to the foetus) even if it fails to prevent pregnancy (which is unlikely if you took it within 72 hours of sex). If you have delayed seeking help a copper intra-uterine device (IUD) can be inserted up to five days after intercourse as an alternative method of emergency contraception.

Breastfeeding and miscarriage

Sometimes longed-for pregnancies end in miscarriage. The signs of miscarriage may be vaginal bleeding and cramps in your lower abdomen. It is common to feel guilty as well as sad. As mothers most of us blame ourselves for everything. Was it because you were still breastfeeding? No. Ongoing breastfeeding and the release of oxytocin only affect pregnancies that are already unstable and unlikely to continue to term. You may need to take painkillers as you would for period pains. Sometimes not all the 'products of conception' may be expelled – that's the technical description, upsetting as it may sound. You may need an operation to make sure the womb is clear, or you may be given the same drugs as you would for a termination. In either case you can still breastfeed. The anaesthetic will not affect your nursling. You may be offered a two-stage medication procedure: a mifepristone 200mg tablet orally, followed 24–48 hours later by misoprostol 800 micrograms. This is usually given as a pessary, but can be a tablet under the tongue. You may also be given painkillers and antibiotics. To be on the safe side you can breastfeed as normal after the mifepristone, but wait four hours after the misoprostol to avoid any risk of diarrhoea in the breastfeeding baby. Give yourself time to grieve – this was the loss of a dream as well as a baby. Many families don't share the news of a pregnancy until after the 12-week scan 'just in case', but if something happens you need friends to care for you, so consider letting them know what's happened.

Prevention of recurrent miscarriage

Some women experience recurrent miscarriages and need

to take medication in order to protect the foetus. This may include the use of 75mg aspirin and progesterone pessaries. Both of these are compatible with continuing to breastfeed an older child. We avoid the use of aspirin at an analgesic dose (600mg four times a day) because of the possible risk of inducing Reye's syndrome and because we have good, effective alternatives such as paracetamol and ibuprofen. There are no recorded cases linking Reye's syndrome with the amount of aspirin passing through breastmilk at a dose of 75mg a day.

Reye's is a rare syndrome, characterised by acute encephalopathy (inflammation of the brain) and fatty degeneration of the liver, usually after a viral illness or chickenpox. The incidence is falling but sporadic cases are still reported. It was often associated with the use of aspirin during the period preceding full symptoms of illness. Few cases occur in white children under one year old, although it is more common in black infants in this age group. Many children retrospectively examined show an underlying inborn error of metabolism.

Progesterone (Cyclogest) used as a pessary or suppository passes into breastmilk at very low levels and does not impact on the baby or milk supply.

Breastfeeding if you decide you need to terminate a pregnancy

Some mothers find themselves pregnant unexpectedly and in such circumstances that they feel that they cannot continue with the pregnancy. In this situation you may be offered a surgical termination. You can breastfeed as normal after this as the amount of anaesthetic in breastmilk will not affect your nursling. You may also be offered a two-stage medication procedure: a mifepristone 200mg tablet orally, followed 24–48 hours later by misoprostol 800 micrograms. This is usually given as a pessary, but can be a tablet under the tongue. You may also be given painkillers and antibiotics. To be on the safe side you can breastfeed as normal after the mifepristone, but wait four hours after the misoprostol to avoid any risk of diarrhoea in the breastfeeding baby.

Withdrawal from drugs used in pregnancy

Some drugs produce symptoms of withdrawal when they are stopped. Examples include venlafaxine, fluoxetine and paroxetine. For babies exposed in the womb there can be a difficult period in the first week before they adapt to the lower level in breastmilk. Some authorities suggest that mothers who have taken these drugs should remain in hospital in order to keep the baby under observation; others do not. If you have taken fluoxetine, venlafaxine or paroxetine in pregnancy I recommend that you discuss hand expression with your midwife before the birth, so that if your baby is sleepy and hard to rouse you can stimulate your milk supply and keep the baby's blood sugars up, reducing the risk of it being suggested that you top up with formula milk. It would also be useful to have a plan detailed in your hand-held notes, recording that it has been confirmed that you can breastfeed on the medication and that you understand the need to seek urgent medical support if your baby stops passing urine and appropriate colour poo (meconium [dark green bowel motions] turning to yellow by day 5).

Fluoxetine is one of the safest of the antidepressants used in pregnancy and although ideally it would be best to switch to a drug with a shorter half-life during the first six weeks after birth, this is often not possible. Where the mother's symptoms are well controlled it would be unfortunate to destabilise her at the most vulnerable period. In the first week after delivery the baby may be very sleepy. Some babies, however, behave perfectly normally and there is no way of determining how a baby will react. If the drowsiness is unexpected it may lead to panic, and in one case I know of admission to special care. After a week even the sleepiest babies seem to become alert and behave normally. It is thought that this behaviour is due to the long half-life of the drug, and the baby's immature kidneys and liver taking time to clear it. Neonatal withdrawal and toxicity have been reported in pre-term infants, but are believed to be due to in-utero exposure rather than breastmilk levels (Hale online, accessed April 2016).

One mother had been taking fluoxetine 40mg throughout pregnancy and continued after the birth. At her six-week check the receptionist informed her that the GP had refused to issue any more repeats for the drug, and had decided (without consulting the mother) to switch the drug to sertraline. The mother had suffered with symptoms of Obsessive Compulsive Disorder (OCD) for eight years, but had been well controlled for some time. Being refused her medication made her anxious. The baby had shown no signs of adverse effects; no colic, irritability or poor weight gain. He was thriving on breastmilk and his mother was enjoying feeding him. However, faced with the switch of drugs she was preparing to stop breastfeeding. Her only concern was whether the baby would experience any withdrawal from the fluoxetine he had been exposed to through breastmilk. She was frustrated that the consultants she had seen in pregnancy, the midwives and the health visitors had shown no concerns about the medication during pregnancy or breastfeeding. To be informed that she couldn't have more medication by the receptionist felt unfair and rude. I provided her with information on the risks of the drugs in breastfeeding a six-week-old (or rather lack of them) and she decided to contact the GP to request a further supply of fluoxetine and to continue breastfeeding.

Babies exposed to paroxetine in utero have demonstrated symptoms of neonatal withdrawal syndrome (Hudak, 2012). Symptoms may include crying, irritability, poor suck or feeding difficulties, tremor, hypoglycaemia (low blood sugar) and, very rarely, seizures. As with fluoxetine, hand expression may help if the baby has hypoglycaemia and poor suck initially.

Venlafaxine is a serotonin and noradrenaline reuptake inhibitor used for severe depression that hasn't responded to other drugs. Infants exposed in utero may have adverse effects immediately at birth, including respiratory distress, difficulty breathing, seizures and temperature instability. It is not known if these are due to a direct toxic effect of venlafaxine on the foetus, or to a discontinuation (withdrawal) syndrome. Studies (Koren, 2006) have shown that adverse effects may be partially relieved by the venlafaxine received through breastmilk. Infants receive venlafaxine and its active metabolite in breastmilk, and the metabolite of the drug can be found in the plasma of most breastfed infants, but no proven drug-related side-effects have been reported (LactMed).

Babies exposed to beta-blockers in pregnancy and during the postnatal period experience different effects. These drugs are usually prescribed to mothers who have developed symptoms of pre-eclampsia, including high blood pressure. The impact of this condition means that babies are often born 'small for dates', or suffering from intra-uterine growth retardation (IUGR). Labour may be induced before the due date so that maternal symptoms can be halted before there is serious damage or symptoms of eclampsia develop, which can be fatal for mother and baby. In all circumstances babies are born vulnerable. Beta-blockers are also known to affect blood glucose levels. So we have a small baby who hasn't been well nourished due to restricted blood supply via the placenta, and already at risk of low blood sugars. Drugs like labetolol and propranolol get into milk in very low levels, so are unlikely to further impact on blood sugars in the baby. However, in most units any baby being breastfed by a mother on beta-blockers is subject to a hypoglycaemia policy, which may mean frequent heel-pricks to check blood sugars. Frequent, effective breastfeeding to stimulate a good milk supply in the mother is hugely important. Even a small volume of colostrum can boost blood sugars considerably and remove the need for formula supplements.

Tandem feeding

Each of the situations discussed above involves the mother, a foetus or newborn and an older breastfed sibling. Tandem feeding may not be well understood by healthcare professionals, and comments such as 'the older baby will take all the goodness from the new baby' are not uncommon. Remember that the decisions about how you feed your babies are yours and yours alone. One useful way of dealing with unwelcome comments may be to smile sweetly, thank the person for their help, then do exactly what you want! Being angry, while totally natural, can spoil your day and your time with your family. Other people's thoughts and beliefs are their own. They do not need to become yours. If the comments come from your own family or in-laws it can be very difficult. You may feel that you need to defend your choices, and it may lead to arguments and even tears, but please try not to let it destroy relationships.

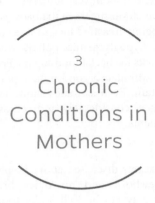

3

Chronic
Conditions in
Mothers

Many women now become pregnant, give birth and breastfeed despite having chronic medical conditions that need ongoing medication. Ideally a treatment plan should be drawn up during pregnancy, with input from midwives, obstetricians and paediatricians, as well as the specialists responsible for the mother's health and the mother herself. Getting all of these people to agree might be a challenge! There is a need to balance the risk to the mum and baby of not breastfeeding with the risk to the baby of receiving breastmilk containing the mother's medication.

Prescribing for a breastfeeding mother is a unique situation as it affects another person who does not need treating – the nursing baby. The incidence of adverse events in the baby definitely attributable to the passage of a drug through the mother's breastmilk is much lower than we might expect. In 2003 Phil Anderson (who was responsible for setting up LactMed) conducted a search for all published studies and case reports on adverse events in infants caused by medications (excluding drugs of abuse) in breastmilk. He identified 100 case reports. Using a standard ranking scale, none were considered to be 'definite', 47% were 'probable' and 53% were 'possible'. Drugs with central nervous system activity accounted for half of all reports. Three reported fatalities involved central nervous system depressants, but each had extenuating circumstances (previous near-miss SIDS; signs of neglect, identified at post mortem, by a mother on methadone; overlaying by mother on phenobarbitone, an old-fashioned sleeping tablet). At least 63% of reported cases were in neonates and 78% were in infants two months or younger; only 4% of adverse reactions occurred in infants older than six months of age. Perversely, it is often mothers of older babies who are advised to stop breastfeeding, and multiple drugs are often prescribed in the neonatal period. Anderson's conclusion was that *Medication use during breastfeeding shortens the duration of breastfeeding often because of overly cautious information given by healthcare providers*.

A systematic review (Saha et al, 2015) looked at postpartum women's use of medication and the effect on breastfeeding. They acknowledged that the need to take medication is one of women's self-reported reasons for discontinuing breastfeeding, while many healthcare professionals lack evidence-based knowledge and advise women to stop breastfeeding unnecessarily. This reflects my professional experience. All of the studies reviewed (except one) suggested that more than 50% of women required medication during the post-partum period, while one hospital-based study reported that this was as high as 100% if vitamins and minerals were included. The most commonly used drugs were analgesics, antibiotics and anti-inflammatory drugs. One study (Matheson, 1990) found that women were more doubtful about medication use during breastfeeding than during pregnancy. One explanation for this may be the widespread belief that we have a 'safe' alternative to feed babies (formula milk). However, the evidence is very clear that formula can never come close to replicating breastmilk, so perhaps we should be researching why we overlook the importance of breastmilk so readily.

When I think about what I want doctors to know about breastfeeding and the safety of drugs in breastmilk, it boils down to this:

- How to signpost to a local breastfeeding specialist
- How to access databases and expert books on the safety of drugs in breastmilk

In the rest of this chapter I present some case studies of mothers with chronic conditions who have breastfed despite needing medication (names and situations have been altered to preserve anonymity).

Rheumatoid arthritis

Sonia told me that she had not been able to feed her first baby. She had suffered with rheumatoid arthritis (RA) since her early 20s and had been stabilised prior to getting pregnant on Etanercept (Enbrel) which she had injected twice weekly. Etanercept is an anti-TNF (tumour necrosis factor) drug. She had a caesarean at 34 weeks and had a little boy weighing 4lb 10oz. The baby was put to the breast while she was in recovery, but in her words 'I had nothing to give him', so she agreed to give him a formula feed and then to carry on formula feeding, as she had been told by her nurse specialist that she could only breastfeed for a short time before recommencing the injections. Now pregnant again, she sought information about breastfeeding, at least initially, as the same nurse specialist had told her that breastfeeding offers some protection to the mother from worsening symptoms of RA. She had also read on the internet that mothers in the USA were allowed to have treatment and continue to breastfeed.

RA is a painful autoimmune disease which produces swelling and pain in the joints, restricting movement. Treatments fall into three categories:

- Painkillers – paracetamol and non-steroidal anti-inflammatory drugs (ibuprofen, naproxen, diclofenac) with the addition of drugs such as codeine and tramadol as needed
- Disease-modifying anti-rheumatic agents (DMARDS), which slow down the development of the disease: azathioprine, gold injections (not possible to use during breastfeeding), hydroxychloroquine, leflunomide, methotrexate (not possible to use during breastfeeding), and sulfasalazine
- Steroids – may be injected into the joints or given as oral prednisolone

Lots of these options are breastfeeding friendly. There is indeed research showing that breastfeeding – particularly for longer than 12 months – reduces the risk of developing RA.

Etanercept has been studied, but in relatively few mothers, just two of whom were breastfeeding. No drug was found in either baby's bloodstream. The drug has a very large molecular weight (150,000 Daltons) and so is most unlikely to pass into milk at all. In addition it has zero bioavailability (none can be absorbed from the gut), so even if some drug did pass into milk the baby would be unable to absorb it so none would transfer into the bloodstream.

I was thus able to tell Sonia that breastfeeding might help to protect her own health, as well as that of her baby. As with many other auto-immune diseases breastfeeding is protective for the baby, preventing foreign proteins from passing through the gut wall and triggering a reaction. She could take painkillers, apply topical anti-inflammatory gels, have oral prednisolone up to 40mg a day and use Etanarcept to reduce the progress of the condition, all while breastfeeding.

Depression

The 'baby blues' affects about 80% of mothers in the first three to five days after delivery and most women soon feel better. However, for some mothers it progresses to ongoing postnatal depression, which sucks the joy out of life. It may be accompanied by sleep changes (sleeping more or less), and variations in appetite (not wanting to eat or munching on everything). Symptoms may persist for weeks and months, and may be accompanied by feelings of exhaustion and lack of interest in sex (although this is common among sleep-deprived mothers!). Depression can also begin suddenly several months after birth.

Amanda had been feeling low for many months. She had been to see her doctor but had been told that she couldn't have any medication unless she stopped breastfeeding. He gave her a referral for Cognitive Behavioural Therapy (CBT) with the local mental health team, but when she spoke to them she was told that there was a waiting list of at least three months, even though as a mother with a baby under one she would be seen as a priority. Further, they also told her that she would have to leave her baby elsewhere during the CBT sessions, as the negative atmosphere in the therapy room might be harmful to the baby's development. All this deterred Amanda from seeking treatment. After several more months she reached a point where she felt that she had to do something. She asked if there was medication that could dry up her milk supply. She had tried weaning her baby from the breast, but when her baby cried she found it heartbreaking and put the baby back to the breast.

I was able to provide Amanda with information to take back to her doctor suggesting that she be prescribed sertraline 50mg to be taken every morning. I reassured Amanda and her doctor that there was minimal transfer into milk and that it was safe for the baby as well as effective. Amanda had never taken an antidepressant before. If she had I would have provided information on the safety of that drug. If possible I prefer to avoid fluoxetine in the first six weeks after delivery because of the long half-life (see page 50). However, if fluoxetine works for a particular mother I would still support her to take it and continue breastfeeding, while cautioning her to watch for colic, irritability or drowsiness in the baby.

As far as access to CBT is concerned, sadly demand is outstripping availability. I asked my daughter, a CBT therapist, why Amanda had been told that her baby (who would be 10 months old) could not be in the therapy room. She explained that rather than the therapy traumatising or harming the baby, Amanda might not be able to give her full attention to what can be a challenging process. In an ideal world the CBT service provides somewhere safe to leave the baby with a trusted person. If the mother has no one to stay with the baby, a healthcare worker might be able to babysit for the period of the appointment. My daughter also says that as a therapist it is very difficult to ignore a baby, whether crying or smiling. In her practice she tries to offer telephone support as an option, although this is generally less effective. Sadly, if you are feeling depressed, being separated from your baby, even for an hour, can add to the stress of the situation. If you have no relatives or close friends and your partner is not around in the daytime it can make you feel more isolated.

There is another factor to consider in depression and breastfeeding. A paper published in 2015 (Borra, 2015) showed that breastfeeding was protective against depression when the mother felt that she had succeeded in meeting her own goals. The study of 1,000 women in the UK and Spain showed that mothers who planned to breastfeed and who actually went on to breastfeed for as long as they wished, were around 50% less likely to become depressed than mothers who had not planned to, and who did not, breastfeed. Mothers who planned to breastfeed, but who did not go on to breastfeed, were over twice as likely to become depressed as mothers who had not planned to, and who did not, breastfeed. This underlines the need for good breastfeeding support.

Depression in a mother is not a reason to wean from the breast, and doing so can add hormomal changes to the mix and the probable return of periods. For many women breastfeeding is something they feel positive about. Furthermore, being told to do anything creates a feeling of disempowerment, which may make depression worse.

MRI and CT Scans

I am often asked about MRI and CT scans for breastfeeding mothers. It seems that most hospitals have guidelines that say breastfeeding mothers should stop breastfeeding for 24 hours.

I was interested to read the phrasing of the American College of Radiology (ACR) guideline, which states:

'For all IV iodinated contrast and gadolinium, contrast administration to the mother is considered safe for both the baby and nursing mother.'

However, it goes on to say:

'Mothers who are breastfeeding should be given the opportunity to make an informed decision as to whether to continue or temporarily abstain from breastfeeding

after receiving IV contrast. If the mother remains concerned about any potential ill effects to the infant, she may abstain from breast-feeding for 24 hours with active expression and discarding of breast milk from both breasts during that period. In anticipation of this, she may wish to use a breast pump to obtain milk before the contrast study to feed the infant during the 24-hour period following the examination.'

This seems to me to be open to interpretation by the radiographer depending on how supportive of breastfeeding they are.

The Royal College of Radiologists' guideline states that:

'A very small percentage of the injected dose enters the breastmilk and virtually none is absorbed from the normal gut and no special precautions or cessation of breastfeeding is required' (citing Webb, 2005)

It goes on:

'Discontinue breastfeeding for 24 hours after use of a high-risk agent. The decision on whether to continue or suspend breastfeeding after use of a medium-risk or low-risk agent should be at your discretion in consultation with the mother.' (This is adapted from the MHRA recommendations 2007, a document which has been archived and I haven't been able to access.)

Since the oral bioavailability of gadolinium, the contrast used in MRI, is only 0.8%, and its half-life is 1.7 hours, meaning that it has all gone from the body after 8.5 hours, why should breastfeeding be disrupted for 24 hours?

I have talked to several mothers who have refused to undergo the procedure if they could not breastfeed as normal, or who postponed it until they had pumped enough breastmilk to feed the baby for 24 hours. Cancellation of appointments is both costly to the NHS and distressing for the mother and her family. Any investigation is stressful and anxiety provoking.

Having examined all the studies, I have concluded that MRI scans with and without gadolinium contrast can be undertaken by breastfeeding mothers without interruption to feeding.

CT scans can also be carried out. A variety of contrast agents seem to be used, but the ingredients are largely based on Iohexol and Diatrizoate (using a variety of brand names). Both the American College of Radiology (ACR) and the European Society of Urogenital Radiology note that the available data suggest that it is safe to continue breastfeeding after receiving intravenous contrast. Sadly this is not reflected in local guidelines. Even when mothers have taken in research evidence from Hale and LactMed, their views are dismissed, and on more than one occasion a healthcare professional has refused to conduct the investigation unless the mother signs a form undertaking not to breastfeed for the advised time.

Pain

We all experience pain and it is said that people's perception of pain differs. Some people are much more reluctant to take painkillers than others. There has been research (Sale, 2006) showing that some believe that if you take medication too readily you will become 'immune' and need stronger and stronger drugs. There is no evidence that this is true, except with drugs to which you can become addicted. This includes two common drugs: codeine and tramadol. Taking these regularly for just two weeks can lead to withdrawal when you stop, or to an addiction. I have had contact with mothers who admitted regularly purchasing codeine over the counter from different pharmacies and taking more than the recommended dose.

In the USA it is not possible to purchase codeine over the counter, but it is prescribed as Tylenol 2 and 3. In America hydrocodone (Vicodin) and oxycodone, often prescribed with acetaminophen (Perocet), are used more often than in the UK.

Concern over the use of codeine by breastfeeding mothers has followed an adverse event report from Canada, where a breastfed baby died at 12 days of age. The post-mortem found very high levels of morphine in his blood, because his mother had multiple copies of the gene that changes codeine into morphine, and was taking high-dose co-codamol for episiotomy pain. The mother had reported constipation and sleepiness in herself. She had sought medical help on several occasions prior to the baby's death, as he was lethargic and had intermittent periods of difficulty in breastfeeding (Koren, 2006).

Another study found that ultra-rapid metabolisers chose to take less codeine than their counterparts, complaining of dizziness and constipation (VanderVaart, 2011). They chose to take paracetamol (acetaminophen) and naproxen, or naproxen alone, which were options in the study protocol.

The MHRA (the Government agency monitoring drug adverse effects) has reported that at least 44 cases of neonatal respiratory depression in breastfed infants of codeine-using mothers have been published (MHRA, 2015).

If codeine is taken by a breastfeeding mother she should observe the baby for sedation, and if he becomes drowsy, stop taking the drug at once. Branded products include Tylenol 3 and 4, Solpadeine, Ultramol and Paracodol. Codeine is also a constituent of a wide variety of preparations available over the counter, which contain multiple analgesic ingredients (e.g. Veganin, Feminax, Syndol, Propain, Paramol and Migraleve).

Many mothers are told that their options for pain relief are limited because they are breastfeeding. This really isn't true. The problem is that clinicians do not know which databases to consult and may lack the in-depth knowledge and confidence to prescribe.

Non-steroidal anti-inflammatory drugs (NSAIDs) can be used during breastfeeding. These include ibuprofen (Nurofen), diclofenac (Voltarol, Difene), or naproxen (Naprosyn). These can be taken as tablets or capsules or applied as gels and creams (Fenbid, Phorpain, Ibuleve, Voltarol). NSAIDs can be taken with paracetamol as well.

We try to avoid opiate drugs (those which are usually changed into morphine or morphine-like drugs) as they can make the baby drowsy as well as causing constipation for mum. This family of drugs includes codeine and dihydrocodeine. Tramadol passes into milk in low quantities, but can make mums feel spaced out and nauseous, and is potentially addictive.

If an opiate is needed dihydrocodeine is regarded as safer than codeine, as the metabolism is more predictable and the risk of high levels of morphine in breastmilk due to ultra-rapid metabolism by the mother less likely.

Tramadol (Zamadol, Zydol) is a new type of drug which resembles morphine, but was thought to be less addictive. It is a stronger pain medication. Small amounts of tramadol are secreted into breastmilk. One study of 75 women (Salman, 2011) showed no adverse effects in breastfed infants whose mothers had taken it. As with other opiate painkillers, it is wise to observe the baby for drowsiness, feeding difficulties and breathing problems. If any of these are noted, the drug should be discontinued and medical advice sought immediately.

There are lots of painkillers that allow a breastfeeding mother to continue to feed and be pain free. No one should be left to suffer.

Migraine

Annabelle had a history of migraines but hadn't had one since before she was pregnant. She recognised all the warning signs: nausea, everything looking slightly fuzzy (her description of an aura), sensitivity to light. She had called her GP but was only able to get a telephone consultation. The GP confirmed that it sounded like a migraine, but said that as she was breastfeeding all she could take was paracetamol and ibuprofen. From experience Annabelle knew this wouldn't help. In her medicine cabinet she had sumatriptan 50mg tablets, her normal go-to pain relief in these circumstances. The patient information leaflet in the box said that breastfeeding mothers should express and dump their milk for 12 hours after taking them. That sounded as difficult to deal with as the pain! She struggled into her local pharmacy where she was offered Migraleve, but the pharmacist said he wasn't sure about using it if she was breastfeeding and that it was her choice whether she took it or not.

Sumatriptan is poorly absorbed from the gut, and research has shown that even after injections little gets into milk. The 12 hours pumping and dumping recommended by the manufacturer is the time it takes to be completely removed from the mother's body (using this guideline ensures the manufacturer need not conduct studies or accept responsibility for use during breastfeeding). I have spoken to countless mums over the past 20 years who have taken sumatriptan and continued to breastfeed as normal and no one has reported any effects in their baby. There is no research on the other drugs in this family either (zolmitriptan (Zomig), rizatriptan (Maxalt), almotriptan (Almogran) and naratriptan (Naramig), but it is likely that they all behave in the same way. Formulations that melt in the mouth (are absorbed sub-lingually, under the tongue) are more effective, which confirms that they are poorly absorbed from the gut and unlikely to reach high levels in milk.

Migraleve comes in two forms: yellow, to be taken at the first sign of a migraine, containing a drug to reduce nausea, paracetamol and codeine, and pink, taken later, which is co-codamol. There are concerns about drowsiness with codeine (see Pain, above).

Annabelle could take sumatriptan or Migraleve if she needed, while keeping an eye on her baby for drowsiness. I also have a home remedy that I have found works well for me and for many migraine sufferers I have spoken to over the years. At the first sign of a migraine take a travel sickness remedy of your choice – cinnarazine or hyoscine work well – then 20 minutes later take two paracetamol tablets and 400mg ibuprofen. The travel sickness remedy settles the stomach and allows the body to absorb the painkillers more effectively.

Other prescription options include Paramax (paracetamol and metoclopramide). There are several over-the-counter remedies that claim to relieve symptoms of migraine, including Syndol (paracetamol, codeine and caffeine), Solpadeine Migraine (ibuprofen and codeine), Nurofen tension headache (ibuprofen), Boots Cooling Headache and Migraine Pads, Kool 'n' Soothe Migraine Sheets and 4head Quickstrip. For those suffering frequent migraines preventative treatment such as propranolol may be useful.

Excessive or frequent use of treatments for migraine is associated with medication-overuse headache (headache, which may be daily), so frequent use of these medicines, even at recommended doses, needs careful management. The treatment for medication-overuse headache is to stop all medications. For a week or so headaches and migraines may be more frequent and worse, they will then return to being less frequent. Ten days a month or more of triptan or opiate use is considered to be overuse, whereas fifteen days or more a month of paracetamol (alone) or NSAID use is considered overuse.

Asthma

Amelia asked if she could continue to breastfeed her six-month-old baby while taking 40mg prednisolone daily for a severe asthma exacerbation. I confirmed that she could without harming her nursling and asked if her asthma was usually well controlled with her inhalers. She admitted that she had stopped using her 'preventer' inhaler because she didn't want to expose her baby to the steroid, and she was upset that she now had to use even more as she was struggling to breathe, let alone cope with her baby.

Asthma inhalers, both relievers e.g. salbutamol (Ventolin, Salamol Asmanex), budesonide (Pulmicort) and preventers e.g. beclometasone (Becotide, Qvar, Asmabec, Clenil), fluticasone (Flixotide) or combination inhalers (Symbicort, Fostair, Seretide) work locally in the lungs to control the symptoms of asthma and very low levels reach breastmilk. There is no reason to restrict their use during breastfeeding.

If there is an exacerbation then prednisolone is frequently prescribed to resolve symptoms. Doses of 40mg (eight tablets a day) are usually prescribed, but sometimes higher doses are needed for a little while. This is known to be safe, although long term very high doses present a theoretical need to monitor growth and development, although there is a lack of research as it is such a rare scenario.

Sometimes mothers with allergic asthma, or where symptoms are triggered by exercise, may be prescribed montelukast (Singulair). There is no research on the amount that gets into milk, but this is a drug which is widely prescribed for children. The adult dose is 10mg daily, while a paediatric dose from the age of six months is 4mg. The dose passing through breastmilk is not likely to approach this level.

Amelia was reassured that she could get on top of her current difficulties and return to controlling symptoms with her usual inhalers and medication.

Constipation after a caesarean section

After a caesarean section most mothers have some doses of morphine, possibly as Oramorph liquid, or dihydrocodeine as they have undergone abdominal surgery. All opiates (morphine-type drugs) have a tendency to produce constipation. It may be recommended that mothers take bulk-forming or osmotic laxatives such as lactulose, Fybogel or Movicol to ensure that motions are soft when passed. Stimulant laxatives such as senna (Sennokot) or bisacodyl (Dulcolax) can be taken, but may empty the bowel, which takes several days to refill to produce natural bowel motions.

Eczema

Women often email me in the late stages of pregnancy concerned about how they will deal with the itching and dry skin of eczema. Melanie was troubled about the dry skin she frequently had on her breasts and nipples. She was concerned that her nipples would crack more than usual and this had been reinforced by her midwife, who had suggested that she might not be able to breastfeed. Many symptoms of eczema resolve with adequate moisturising and there is no need to change the formulation normally used because of breastfeeding. Melanie was scared that if she applied anything to her nipples her baby would ingest the chemical and become ill. In fact absorption of all topical preparations is poor and if applied sparingly after feeds even application to the nipples does not cause a problem. Melanie was reassured that she could continue to use the Diprobase cream she used all over her body as a moisturiser and soap substitute. I advised her to keep her nipples supple, but not soggy, and to apply the corticosteroid product she needed as normal over the rest of her body but sparingly and after feeds if she needed to soothe her nipples. I advised her that there was no need to purchase any of the particular products marketed for application to the nipples. She discussed this approach with her midwife at her next routine visit. She emailed me after she had her baby and was delighted to say that she had experienced no soreness, let alone cracking, as she had received excellent breastfeeding support in hospital from the very first feed. She had also tried applying expressed breastmilk to the skin behind her knees, where her eczema often flared, with excellent results.

Psoriasis

Psoriasis is a long-term condition causing scaling of the skin. It appears as red, raised scaly patches known as plaques. These most commonly appear on the elbows, knees and scalp. Ten to 20 per cent of people with psoriasis develop psoriatic arthritis, which causes pain and swelling in the joints. It can also be associated with chronic fatigue. Many mothers ask about the safety of the application of calcipotriene (Dovonex), which is derived from vitamin D. Research cited by Lactmed suggests that although 'No information is available on the use of calcipotriene during breastfeeding. Because it is poorly absorbed after topical application, calcipotriene is probably a low risk to the nursing infant and is generally considered acceptable during breastfeeding, even to the nipple area'.

Suzanne was distraught having been told by her consultant that she was to be prescribed methotrexate to treat her psoriatic arthritis. She was in considerable pain, which wasn't relieved by simple painkillers or the application of non-steroidal gels. Methotrexate is not compatible with breastfeeding.

Disease-modifying anti-rheumatic drugs (DMARDS) including methotrexate are often prescribed in addition to ibuprofen-type drugs to help slow down the processes that cause the chronic inflammation. Other DMARDS include azathioprine, sulfasalazine and hydroxychloroquine, which can be used during breastfeeding.

Corticosteroids as injections into joints can be very effective, but not in all individuals. A group of specialised drugs are also increasingly used including anti-TNF (tumour necrosis factor) drugs such as Infliximab (Remicade) and adalimumab (Humira), which may be offered if other DMARDS have proved ineffective. These drugs are poorly absorbed from the gut and therefore have to be given by injection. They have high molecular weights, which dramatically limit the amounts that pass into breastmilk, making them an option for breastfeeding mothers.

Suzanne returned to her specialist to discuss these other options. He agreed to prescribe an alternative, allowing Suzanne to continue to breastfeed. She breastfed her daughter for two years.

Anxiety

Having a baby is exciting and emotional, but it can also be accompanied by anxiety. Anxiety about getting everything right is normal, but too much anxiety can interfere with our ability to cope with daily activities and enjoy life. Anxiety is more common than depression after birth. It affects 1 in 6 mothers (1 in 5 first-time mums), but is often not as well recognised as depression.

Signs of anxiety include:

- Trouble concentrating and remembering things
- Difficulty finishing everyday tasks

- Trouble making decisions
- Difficulty relaxing
- Insomnia
- Exhaustion
- Feelings of extreme uneasiness for prolonged periods of time
- Loss of appetite
- Possible suicidal thoughts
- Anxiety/panic attacks

Anxious mothers often experience extreme concern about using any medication (sometimes even paracetamol), because it might harm the baby in the future. Mothers also often have problems sleeping, even when the baby has gone back to sleep after waking at night. Mothers lie awake, exhausted but unable to turn off, often experiencing palpitations (the heart beating rapidly), which can make them feel as if they are about to have a heart attack. It is scary, lonely and exhausting. Medications can be prescribed, including propranolol to calm the racing heart and SSRI antidepressants (sertraline, citalopram, fluoxetine or paroxetine). These drugs have both anti-anxiety and antidepressant activity. Mothers often ask 'how can you be sure that taking these drugs will not damage my baby's brain for the future?' There is no reason to believe that the small amount of the drugs passing into breastmilk will do harm to the baby, either in the short term or in the future.

Other treatment options use cognitive behavioural therapy (CBT) to help change the focus of thoughts. These can be accessed through local mental health teams, notably IAPT (Improved Access to Psychological Therapy), but there may be some delay as demand continues to exceed availability.

Mothers often buy products over the counter, such as Kalms, Quiet Life, Bach Flower Remedies, homeopathic remedies and herbal remedies, in an attempt to manage their anxiety. For many plucking up the courage to seek medical help is very difficult. Fear that they may be told to stop breastfeeding prevents women seeking treatment. In a 2013 report 40% of women reporting mental health problems felt that isolation contributed to their feelings, but that often going out proved to be difficult if not impossible. Sadly, 34% of those who had hidden their feelings did so because they were fearful that their baby would be taken away by social services, and 22% admitted to having suicidal thoughts.

Lives are blighted and irreplaceable time with a new baby is lost when mothers feel unable to seek help with their anxiety. Another report, published by the RCGP (Royal College of General Practitioners) in 2015, stated:

> 'A few women stated that they had been "refused" medication by GPs due to their pregnancy and breastfeeding. In these circumstances, there was no mention of any risk/benefit conversation taking place. Neither were women generally offered any other form of support in the absence of this treatment.'

So women who had plucked up courage to call and make an appointment with their GP, had attended and had dared to admit how they felt, were dismissed because they wouldn't give up breastfeeding. This is why mothers' medication matters – these women need compassion and support, as well as urgent treatment.

Other mental health issues

Other mental health problems that affect mothers are less common. One is obsessive compulsive disorder (OCD). Many of us have had some symptoms of OCD at various times. We can become over-particular about hygiene after a bad experience with a tummy bug. After a burglary we might be cautious about house security. If we hear of the tragic death of a child, we may feel desperate to protect our own children. All these are perfectly normal reactions. OCD only becomes a problem when the routines take over our lives and have to be followed multiple times.

Daniel contacted me after leaving his wife in tears. She had an obsession with cleaning the bathroom and toilet. Being admitted to hospital for a caesarean section due to a breech birth was threatening for her. She had her own bathroom attached to her room. The night before the section she scrubbed the bathroom and toilet so she felt reassured that after the birth she and her baby would be relatively safe. However, post-operatively she was taken to a different room. She was in no physical condition to clean the new bathroom and the staff had dismissed her fears, despite knowing her medical history. Daniel did not know how to help. He had to explain to the staff that his wife's fears about contracting an infection from a dirty bathroom were very real. When the shift changed new staff were more sympathetic and allowed the baby's grandmother to visit late in the evening to clean the bathroom. An early discharge was also arranged so that she could settle in her own house.

A second condition that affects some mothers is PTSD (Post-Traumatic Stress Disorder). This can involve flashbacks to a difficult birth, an unexpected caesarean or a post-partum haemorrhage, where staff may have had to act quickly rather than take time to talk though what is happening with the family. In some maternity units midwives are available to discuss what happened at the birth and allow the mother to debrief her experience.

Other PTSD symptoms may include nightmares and

sleep problems. Kelsey was frightened to sleep after the birth of her baby caused a return of fears she thought she had worked through. She was prescribed a sedative antihistamine to help her to sleep, but this caused a hangover effect in the morning, leaving her feeling sluggish for most of the day and still only getting four hours of sleep. She was frightened that she wouldn't hear her baby if he woke during the night. She described her partner as sleeping so deeply that nothing disturbed him, and she felt unable to rely on him to wake her. She was also concerned that the antihistamine would cause her son to be drowsy. He normally fed twice overnight. The dilemmas went round and round – she was exhausted and needed to sleep, but the medication had risks for her too. Her supportive GP managed to arrange some low-intensity CBT for her with immediate effect, bypassing the normal waiting list. This was helpful in her case but sadly doesn't happen for everyone in Kelsey's situation.

I get many questions from mothers who are bipolar. Their medication is often varied according to their current state. Many of them are told that they can continue medication during pregnancy in order to keep their mood stable, but that they will not be able to breastfeed. This seems confusing because the baby has already been exposed to the drug in utero, so why not in breastfeeding? It is true that the baby is exposed to approximately one-tenth of the amount of the drug in breastmilk than is received via the placenta. However, in the womb the drug passes back to the mother's bloodstream to be metabolised, whereas after birth the baby's own kidneys and liver have to detoxify the drug. The kidneys and liver do not reach full maturity for six weeks and may not be able to cope, particularly if the drug has a half-life longer than 24 hours. Nonetheless, the drugs given to treat bipolar disorder can usually be taken during breastfeeding, depending on the dose, so mothers can ask their health professionals to investigate further. An exception is lithium, which is toxic to babies and should be avoided.

Colonoscopy

Colonoscopies require the bowel to be washed out before beginning the procedure. This is accomplished by the use of laxatives, most of which draw water into the bowel to flush faeces out. These osmotic laxatives do not get into breastmilk. The colonoscopy itself is usually performed under conscious sedation, involving the use of a combination of midazolam, pethidine and fentanyl. These drugs have very short half-lives, so mothers are usually wide awake and ready to go home soon after the procedure is over. There is no reason to delay breastfeeding, although many mothers are told they can't breastfeed from when they start the bowel cleanse until 24 hours after the procedure is over. This is not true and breastfeeding can carry on as normal.

Mothers having endoscopies can similarly continue to breastfeed as normal after the sedation, but they do not normally require a bowel washout first.

Inflammatory bowel disease (Crohn's disease and ulcerative colitis)

I have Crohn's disease myself. I was first diagnosed when I was 22 and have had three bowel resections since then. I gave birth to and breastfed all three of my daughters with this chronic condition. However, I was able to time my pregnancies when I had no active symptoms. For me the healthiest years of my life have been when I was pregnant or breastfeeding. It's one reason I became interested in breastfeeding, which led to my work on drugs in breastmilk and ultimately to this book.

Mothers with IBD usually need medication to control their symptoms. These drugs can include prednisolone, azathioprine, mesalamine, infliximab and many of the anti-TNF (tumour necrosis factor) drugs. Many women are told that it is impossible to breastfeed on these drugs. However, it is important that mothers with IBD do breastfeed: those of us with the condition pass on a genetic predisposition to develop it to our children, and it is, at least in part, linked with being formula fed. So it's important that mothers know that they can breastfeed with IBD, even while taking medication, and that there are many advantages to them and their babies of doing so.

Epilepsy

Several of the drugs used to treat epilepsy, such as valproate, carry higher risks of teratogenicity (causing birth defects), so pregnancy planning is essential. In addition, most women with epilepsy who are trying to conceive are advised to take 5mg of folic acid rather than the more common 400mcg, because of the increased risk of neural tube defects. Unplanned pregnancies are not advised.

For some women being pregnant destabilises their epilepsy. Unexpected seizures can be frightening and also have ramifications for everyday life, for example by making driving unsafe. Some mothers are told that they are safer formula feeding so that their sleep is not disturbed, on the assumption that sleep disruption can trigger seizures. I saw some information that suggested that mothers with epilepsy should only feed at night while sitting on the floor, so that in the event of a seizure they were not at risk of smothering their baby on a sofa. This all sounds very scary.

However, most women can have their condition stabilised during pregnancy so that the baby develops well and they remain symptom-free. The dose of some drugs (e.g. lamotrigine) may be increased during pregnancy. Blood levels may need to be monitored after delivery to ensure that they are not too high, and doses may then be changed.

The majority of anti-epilepsy medication can be taken while breastfeeding, with precautionary advice to monitor the baby for drowsiness. The risks of drowsiness increase with the use of more than one medication in the early weeks, as the baby's liver and kidneys mature. Possible drugs include lamotrigine, topiramate and levetiracetam, clobazam, clonazepam, valproate, phenytoin and carbamazepine.

Helen contacted me when pregnant with her third child to ask if more information had become available since the birth of her previous children, whom she had been advised to formula feed, much to her disappointment. On discovering that she could have breastfed them she experienced anger and sadness that none of her specialist team of nurses and doctors had been able to access the evidence and information I was able to show her. She felt that she had let her children down. It took much discussion and listening before she could begin to accept that she had done the best she could with the information she had, and that her team were not to blame for the fact that the information is not more readily available. She decided to work with them to develop information for other mothers locally in the future.

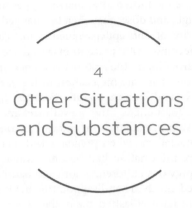

4

Other Situations
and Substances

Perceived breastmilk insufficiency

We know that many women give up breastfeeding sooner than they had intended because they believe that they don't have enough milk. Statistically, only a very few women are unable to produce milk. However, lack of good breastfeeding support in the early days and a delay in establishing breastfeeding can impact on the volume of milk produced.

Emily contacted me when her baby was four weeks old. She had developed pre-eclampsia at 36 weeks and was induced at 38 weeks. Her baby was born vaginally weighing 5lb 6oz. She was prescribed labetolol 200mg three times a day in pregnancy and this was continued postnatally as her blood pressure remained high. On the ward the baby had been drowsy and was offered formula top-ups until Emily's milk came in. Breastfeeding was painful, but she was told that this was normal and that her nipples would soon harden up. They were discharged three days after delivery with Emily giving 30ml top-ups after three feeds a day. Breastfeeding continued to be painful no matter how hard she tried. She went to a drop-in group when her baby was four weeks old and the health visitor noted a tongue-tie. The baby was referred to the tongue-tie clinic, but Emily was told there was a two-week waiting list. As the baby's weight gain was satisfactory (due to the top-ups!) she was not seen as a priority. By this point she was offering top-ups after most feeds, which is why the weight gain seemed satisfactory. She returned to the group the following week and asked for help reducing the total volume of formula she was giving. On discussion she mentioned that her nipples hurt at random times of the day and often when she was cold. She had a history of cold hands and feet in winter, but had never had a diagnosis of Raynaud's syndrome. The health visitor suggested that she visit her GP and ask for a prescription for domperidone 10mg three times a day (to increase her milk supply) and nifedipine 10mg three times a day (to help with the symptoms of Raynaud's). She contacted me to ask if the combination of these drugs on top of the labetolol was suitable for her to carry on breastfeeding.

Having listened to her history I suggested that she ask her GP to switch her labetolol to a different anti-hypertensive which does not cause vasoconstriction, which I felt was precipitating the symptoms of pain when she was cold and the white nipples. I suggested that she be prescribed enalapril, very little of which passes into breastmilk. I hoped that, following the tongue-tie snip and help with breastfeeding, her milk supply would increase without the need for domperidone. The effectiveness of domperidone after five weeks is not supported by research. We discussed the impact of the top-ups and the need for frequent feeding to increase her supply. She returned to her health visitor to discuss using a nursing supplementer to provide the formula rather than a bottle, to help stimulate her breasts during this period.

After two weeks she contacted me to say that she no longer felt pain between feeds and that applying heat straight after a feed had proved sufficient to stop pain after feeding. The baby had taken a few days to settle after the tongue-tie snip but was now feeding more effectively. The volume of supplements had reduced to once a day and Emily was planning to stop that shortly as she felt reassured that her own supply had increased dramatically.

Drinking alcohol

Some young mothers are so concerned that they have to continue to restrict their alcohol intake (the NHS recommendation is to consume no alcohol during pregnancy) that they choose not to breastfeed. However, it is acceptable to drink alcohol while breastfeeding with a few sensible precautions.

- If possible restrict alcohol intake until after the baby has had the last feed of the day (this ignores the fact that most babies will breastfeed overnight – the idea is to leave the longest possible gap between drinking and the baby's next feed)
- Avoid breastfeeding for one hour after each unit of alcohol consumed to avoid exposure of the baby to any alcohol

Most breastfeeding women do not drink significant amounts after nine months of abstinence and while they need to wake regularly during the night to feed the baby. Occasional social drinking of one or two glasses of wine (sensible size glasses!) will not affect the baby. If this was to be continued every day of the week then it would not be healthy for the mother.

If you do decide to go out and drink heavily – to the point of vomiting – then it would not be advisable to breastfeed until the following morning. I would say that you should express and discard your milk to maintain your supply; but if you're that drunk you might not manage it! However, depending on the age of your baby, you may need to express for comfort.

If you have consumed a significant amount of alcohol it is imperative that you *do not co-sleep* with your baby, or fall asleep with them in a chair or on a sofa. This dramatically increases the risk of SIDS (Sudden Infant Death Syndrome, otherwise known as cot death).

Recreational drugs

Emily has a five-month-old daughter. She rang and said that she had acted totally out of character and was bitterly ashamed of herself, having taken cocaine on Saturday evening. She was calling on Monday morning and had been crying all night. She had not breastfed since but was desperate to resume as soon as it was safe to do so.

Cocaine is the second most commonly used illicit drug (second only to cannabis). The prevalence of cocaine use in the UK is documented at 8.9% lifetime use and 0.8% in the previous month, although it is said to be declining (European Monitoring Centre for Drugs and Drug Addiction, 2012; Shannon, 1989). Adverse effects include agitation, nervousness, euphoria, hallucinations, tremors, seizures and changes in heart rhythm. The duration of a high is only 20–30 minutes, but metabolism and excretion take much longer, with urine remaining positive for metabolites for up to seven days. The euphoric effect is usually followed by a crash, leading to the user wanting to take more. Significant amounts pass to breastfeeding infants because it concentrates in breastmilk. A mother may assume that if she now feels 'normal' then the cocaine has left her system and it is safe to breastfeed. This is not true. The baby remains at serious risk from the amount passing through breastmilk for at least 24 hours after the mother last used. She should pump and dump her breastmilk for a period of 72 hours.

Emily was very upset that she could not return to breastfeeding for a further 36 hours, as her baby was not settling well on formula. It was hard to hear her distress (and the sound of her baby crying in the background). As she put it herself, nothing was worth this.

Marijuana (cannabis, weed) seems to be regarded as a relatively harmless drug, producing relaxation and calm. I get more queries about it from healthcare professionals than from mothers. The active component, delta-9-THC (tetrahydrocannabinol), is rapidly distributed to the brain and fat tissue and is stored there for long periods (weeks to months). Small to moderate secretion into breastmilk has been documented.

We have some limited studies, some showing no effects on the breastfed infant and others showing a decrease in motor development, particularly if it is used in the first month after birth. Infants exposed to it will test positive in urine screens for long periods of time (2–3 weeks). Hale suggests the studies show that cannabis use may have long-term consequences for babies, such as reduced cognition and changes in mood and reward. We know that regular users may show symptoms of paranoia. Will young babies exposed via their mother's milk, let alone by passive smoking, show these symptoms as they mature? We do not have the evidence at present, but cannabis use concerns me more than social alcohol consumption and I worry that while we wait for evidence babies' brains will be permanently altered. It is one of the few occasions when I would say that if a mother smokes cannabis regularly and chronically, the baby may be better off being formula fed.

Threadworms

Mothers with older children at nursery or school often ask

about threadworm treatment. Ovex is the most commonly used form of mebendazole, along with Vermox. The manufacturers state that 'As it is not known whether mebendazole is excreted in human milk, it is not advisable to breastfeed following administration of Ovex'. However, within the prescribing information they also state that 'Following oral administration, approximately <10% of the dose reaches the systemic circulation, due to incomplete absorption and to extensive pre-systemic metabolism (first-pass effect)'. The *BNF* says 'amount in breastmilk too small to be harmful but manufacturer advises avoid'. Hale (online, accessed August 2016) confirms that '*Considering the poor oral absorption and high protein binding, it is unlikely that mebendazole would be transmitted to the infant in clinically relevant concentrations*'. Despite this, most mothers are told to avoid breastfeeding for eight hours after taking mebendazole. This is totally unnecessary.

Operations

There are many reasons why a breastfeeding mother may need to have an operation under general anaesthetic. Julie contacted me about the removal of gallstones.

Julie, as in almost every case, had been told at her pre-op assessment that she would not be able to breastfeed for 48 hours after surgery due to the administration of the anaesthetic agents. This always confuses me. The drugs used to anaesthetise are almost identical to those used for a mother undergoing a caesarean section under a general anaesthetic. In the latter case the baby may be put to the mother's breast in the recovery room before she is fully conscious! The baby may find its own way to the nipple if left in skin-to-skin contact. At the time of birth the gaps between the cells in the breast are wide open to facilitate the transfer of immunoglobulins to protect the baby. When most women have surgery on their gallbladders their babies are significantly older and these gaps are closed, restricting the passage of most drugs except across the cellular membranes. Anaesthetic drugs such as propofol reach only minimal levels in breastmilk. So why are mothers advised not to breastfeed for 48 hours?

One mother described how the staff she met expressed their disgust (her word) at the fact that she was still breastfeeding an 11-month-old. Another was told by the anaesthetist that a three-month-old would do well on cows' milk and didn't need to be breastfed. These comments are in no way evidence based. Is this acceptable from a healthcare professional? Would similar non-evidence-based comments be made about any other aspect of life? These two mothers chose to complain about their treatment to the hospital involved, which took courage when they needed ongoing medical care.

Anticoagulants and blood clots

Anticoagulant drugs such as the low molecular weight heparins (dalteparin (Fragmin), enoxaparin (Clexane), tinzaparin (Innohep) and heparin itself) are used in any situation where there is a risk of development of a blood clot (after surgery, including after caesarean section). When a clot has developed higher doses are used, with an ongoing lower dose to prevent reoccurrence. (See Chapter 2.)

Warfarin is an oral anticoagulant (taken by mouth as a tablet) that may be used long term. It requires frequent monitoring of blood clotting, but levels in breastmilk are low.

There is no reason to stop breastfeeding when using any of these drugs, despite what the patient information leaflets may suggest.

Podiatry treatment

One simple procedure that seems to cause a lot of controversy is the removal of ingrowing toenails by podiatrists. This involves the use of a local anaesthetic to numb the area so that the ingrowing nail can be cut away. Usually phenol or sodium hydroxide is applied to the affected area to prevent the nail growing back and becoming ingrown in the future. Neither the local anaesthetic nor the small amount of phenol or sodium hydroxide is absorbed into the bloodstream, let alone the milk. Nonetheless, mothers are regularly told not to breastfeed for a minimum of 24 hours, and I have been told of one mother who was told that she could not breastfeed for a week and might as well give up altogether. Others have been refused surgery until they have stopped breastfeeding. Phenol is used in many dental products including toothpastes and mouthwashes, but one podiatrist told a mother that in nail surgery they used a 'different' phenol. Phenol is phenol to this pharmacist!

Dental treatment, including sedation

Two types of question arise about breastfeeding and dental treatment. One is about the mother receiving treatment – fillings, local anaesthetic, extractions, infections and pain. The other comes from mothers who have been told by dentists that their children's teeth have been damaged by long-term breastfeeding, especially night feeds.

Two dentists, Dr Brian Palmer and Dr Harold Torney, conducted research on human skulls (from 500–1,000 years ago) in their study of tooth decay in children. These children would have been breastfed, probably for several years. Their research led them to conclude that breastfeeding does not cause tooth decay. The confusion probably arises because of decay caused by long-term use of bottles containing formula milk or sweetened liquids such as juices. With bottles the milk pools within the mouth, bathing the teeth. However, when breastfeeding the nipple is pulled far back into the baby's mouth and milk flows over the soft palate as the baby sucks. If the baby doesn't suck there is no milk to pool. Dr Torney showed that some breastfed babies do have dental decay, but this is because they have poor enamel on their teeth. Enamel defects occur when the first teeth are forming in the womb before birth, and the decay is not caused by breastfeeding. In fact breastfeeding protects due to the antibodies in breastmilk.

Mothers feel terribly guilty if their children have tooth decay and need to have teeth filled or even extracted. To be told that breastfeeding, which we perceive as the most protective thing we can do for our children, is the cause is devastating, but untrue. However, it is difficult to believe this when a dentist has pointed the finger of responsibility, even when we know what the research has shown. If your baby has not had highly sweetened foods and drinks it is unlikely that you have caused the damage post-natally.

Turning to the treatment of our own teeth, Stephanie's dentist told her that if her mercury filling was removed while she was breastfeeding, her baby would be exposed to a toxic level of mercury, which would be vaporised as it was drilled out. He said that the filling would have to wait until she had finished breastfeeding. Stephanie was a committed long-term breast feeder and pointed out that this might not be for some years, and she was already experiencing pain from the tooth. The dentist raised his eyebrows and sent her away to consider her decision.

The evidence shows that very little mercury is absorbed during the removal process. Most is vaporised and any lumps are removed by the dental assistant using the vacuum suction. We rarely swallow any of the filling. Mercury is around us all the time and our exposure is higher during a walk down the street thanks to car exhausts.

Innumerable other mothers have been concerned about

local anaesthetics passing into breastmilk. We know that locals work very close to the area of injection; for example, an injection to numb the gum does not numb the whole face. The body breaks down the drug close to where it is injected and it does not pass into breastmilk. One mother was told that if she breastfed after having an injection her baby's mouth would become numb! The mother laughed, but later began to worry because a healthcare professional had said this. It is nonsense.

One mother who had several teeth extracted under a general anaesthetic was told she couldn't breastfeed again for a week. (See above, Operations.)

So breastfeeding mothers can have teeth filled and extracted. However, some are very nervous about dental treatment and opt for conscious sedation. This involves the use of a drug, usually midazolam (Versed), which relaxes the patient and also tends to produce amnesia about the treatment so that it becomes less stressful. LactMed reports that two expert panels agree that if midazolam is used on a mother with a baby under two months of age, four hours should be allowed to elapse before continuing breastfeeding as normal. If the baby is more than two months old breastfeeding can continue as normal. Midazolam reaches breastmilk in extremely low concentrations.

Other cosmetic dental procedures include teeth whitening. The baths containing the bleach should not leak, so there should be no absorption into breastmilk. The use of high-strength fluoride toothpastes also appears to present no risk so long as the paste is not swallowed. Absorption via the teeth into milk is unlikely, although there is no research that I have been able to find.

Cosmetic procedures

Whatever the rights and wrongs of our society's obsession with physical beauty, the use of cosmetic products and procedures is often of concern to mothers. I have been asked over the years whether breastfeeding mothers can:

- Have false nails fitted or acrylic nails applied
- Have their hair permed, dyed or straightened
- Have relaxing massages or go to the spa
- Have tattoos – body art or eyebrow tattoos
- Apply anti-wrinkle cream
- Use hair removers or have bikini waxes

The answer to all of these is yes. The proviso with tattoos is to use a reputable artist with good hygiene to avoid infection risk.

I am also asked about Botox. In one area a company offered cut price treatment to new mums! We don't have research on the use of Botox as a cosmetic injection, but we do know that *'one infant was safely breastfed during maternal botulism and no botulinum toxin was detectable in the mother's milk or infant. Since the doses used medically are far lower than those that cause botulism, amounts ingested by the infant, if any, are expected to be insignificant and not cause any adverse effects in breastfed infants.'* (LactMed) I provide this information without comment for you to make your own decision.

Similarly, dermal fillers used in lip augmentation are assumed to be inert, but there is no research into their use during breastfeeding.

Concerns about breast implants are common, especially in the wake of the health scandal that saw many faulty implants rupture. Breast augmentation is less risk to breastfeeding than breast reduction. Surgeons are usually able to place the implant so as not to damage the breast tissue and affect lactation. Some women choose not to breastfeed for fear of damaging their figure, but it is actually pregnancy which causes changes to the breasts, not breastfeeding. Breast reduction surgeons should ask women if they plan to breastfeed in the future, but of course women may respond based on how they feel at that time and later regret their decision. Surgery may result in damage to the milk ducts and re-siting of the nipple. The more nerves are cut, the less likely it is that a mother will be able to breastfeed in the future. Stimulation of the nerves in the nipples is essential for milk production.

Herbs and supplements

I am often asked whether dietary supplements and herbs are compatible with breastfeeding. General vitamin and mineral supplements are suitable as long as they have 10mcg (400 IU) of vitamin D (many only have half this amount, so you may need to take additional vitamin D). They can contain vitamin A at normal (not mega) doses of less than 700µg or 2,300 IU. They should contain folic acid 400mcg in case of accidental pregnancy. You do not need to take supplements specifically aimed at breastfeeding mothers.

Health food store supplements are more problematic. There is often no information about their use while breastfeeding. These supplements are generally regarded as coming under food supplement legislation, and unless they carry a health claim saying that they can relieve the symptoms of a condition they do not need to provide evidence of efficacy or a product licence number (these are required for medicines). Many people are looking for dietary answers to common problems and many women will try these supplements; at the moment we don't have any evidence that they will work or any data about how they might affect breastfeeding or our nursing babies.

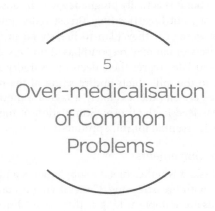

5

Over-medicalisation of Common Problems

Breastfeeding mothers regularly visit their doctors seeking treatment for common conditions. Not all of these need treatment with medication; some can be treated with good information and basic breastfeeding help. Sadly, many doctors have received no training in managing breastfeeding problems, and they have very limited time for appointments. In this situation simple problems can become medicalised and treated with medication that might not otherwise be needed. Ideally, doctors would know when, and how, to refer mothers to named breastfeeding experts or groups locally who have the expertise to support and encourage breastfeeding. Similarly, if these experts identify a problem that requires medication, they should be able to refer back to the medical professionals with recommendations for treatment. This system works in many specialities from physiotherapy to surgery. Why should breastfeeding be different?

Engorgement
Around day three after birth milk production gradually kicks

in. For some mothers this is uncomfortable as the breasts suddenly swell, due to an increase in blood supply as well as the milk production. Sometimes babies find it difficult to feed as they cannot take enough of the breast into the mouth due to the swelling, leading to painful feeding and a fretful baby. Engorgement can be minimised if the baby is allowed unrestricted access to the breast day and night, and is often caused by 'management' of breastfeeding – in other words, trying to space out feeds.

If the baby is having difficulty feeding from the engorged breast, it may be useful to hand express some milk very gently. Alternatively, applying heat with a warm flannel, or immersing the breasts in a bowl of warm water or a hot shower, may soften the swollen tissue.

Some people also recommend a technique called 'reverse pressure softening'. Firmly but gently (not hard enough to cause pain), press inwards towards the chest area using the flat side of both thumbs above and below the nipple. Continue to press around the nipple, one small area at a time. The aim is to make the area just behind the nipple soft enough to help the baby latch on easily.

If milk accumulates in the breast, the negative feedback hormone FIL (Feedback Inhibitor of Lactation) will be produced, leading to a decreased milk supply in the longer term. Discomfort can be eased by taking paracetamol and/ or ibuprofen, but frequent, effective feeding by the baby or pumping is essential.

I have come across situations where engorgement has been treated as mastitis and antibiotics prescribed. A little knowledge of breastfeeding could prevent this.

Mastitis

Mastitis is an inflammation of the breast, which may develop into an infection, but usually doesn't. However, most mothers who experience symptoms and consult their doctor are prescribed antibiotics. This is clearly undesirable when we all know that from a public health standpoint we need to avoid antibiotics unless they are essential, to avoid the development of bacteria resistant to the drugs.

Mastitis generally develops from a blocked duct and/or engorgement. If an area of the breast is not well drained of milk, the excess milk accumulates. This may occur after a knock to an area of the breast, when the ducts in that area may develop a kink. The analogy I have used for many years is of a hosepipe that has been stored in the garage all winter, which may not straighten out immediately in the spring. In some cases some of the breastmilk (in the case of the hose, the water!) may leak out behind the kink. The body tends to attack this milk as a foreign protein, sending additional plasma and leukocytes to the area. This results in swelling, heat and redness: the typical symptoms that precede full-blown mastitis.

Symptoms can also occur if a breastfeed has been missed (if mum and baby are separated, or baby sleeps through a normal feed time). It can also be a sign that the baby is not effectively draining an area of the breast due to less than perfect attachment.

If the mother recognises the first symptoms – which range from a dull ache in an area to severe pain and a hot red lump – feeding frequently with additional drainage using hand expression or a breast pump can resolve symptoms very quickly. The classic drugs that reduce inflammation are the non-steroidal anti-inflammatories (NSAIDs), the best known of which is ibuprofen. So in addition to frequent drainage, taking 400mg ibuprofen three times a day will help to reduce the pain and swelling. Anecdotally, holding the reverse side of an electric toothbrush against the area also helps to break up the lump by applying gentle massage.

Recently I spoke to Rebecca who had just begun her second course of antibiotics for mastitis. She described the lumpy area as being high up on her breast towards her armpit. We discussed using alternative feeding positions to help drainage (with the baby's chin closest to the lump), which she tried, but with difficulty because the affected area was difficult to access with a four-month-old. Rebecca had been told to reduce the frequency of feeds from the affected breast in order not to stimulate the milk supply – precisely the opposite of what the research says. Even with the use of antibiotics frequent drainage helps the milk to flow freely and resolve symptoms faster. She had read that massaging the area would also help to break up the lump. However, to her this meant effectively squeezing the breast behind the area in an attempt to push the blockage through. She described how the swollen area was increasing. I suspect that she had produced a cellulitis in the area, the symptoms of which are not dissimilar to mastitis – redness, swelling and local pain, with the area looking slightly glossy or shiny where the skin is stretched tight. I explained that what she needed to do was *gently* massage across the area to encourage the milk to flow as she fed. I suggested she imagine stroking the most shy and frightened kitten she had ever met. Rebecca had no temperature or shivering, which is common in mastitis, but had been taking both ibuprofen and paracetamol regularly alongside the antibiotics. We discussed what might happen next and decided that if her symptoms began to resolve with frequent drainage and gentle massage we could assume all was well. She also knew what to do if she ever experienced symptoms in the future. However, I was concerned that if the lump did not begin to resolve she might have an abscess. I suggested that she should return to the doctor and ask for a sample of her milk to be cultured, to ensure that the correct antibiotics had been prescribed for the infection she had. Additionally I recommended that she ask her GP to send her for an ultrasound to rule out an abscess (Dixon, 2011).

In general, self-help measures as described to Rebecca should resolve the red, painful area and any increased temperature quite quickly. If symptoms continue to get worse (or do not improve at all) then the prescription of antibiotics is needed. If you feel seriously unwell, dizzy, confused, develop nausea, vomiting or diarrhoea or slurred speech along with the symptoms of mastitis you need to seek urgent medical attention. These can be signs that mastitis is developing into sepsis. If severe, this is a medical emergency that needs urgent hospital admission and IV antibiotics. This is a rare situation but one that everyone should be aware of.

Thrush

Nineteen years ago, a colleague and I began research into a condition we had both encountered, though rarely, as breastfeeding supporters. This was a collection of symptoms, which were referenced in the literature but not well understood. Mothers would suddenly describe symptoms of agonising pain after feeds after months of pain-free, trouble-free breastfeeding. In almost all cases the mothers had given up breastfeeding in the absence of any solution. We found the description of thrush of the nipples and a very limited amount of information on how to treat this medically.

We published a leaflet describing the symptoms and the treatment, which needed to be prescribed along with self-help measures. Many times since I have regretted that first leaflet. I know that it has rescued breastfeeding for some, but it has also led to over-medicalisation on a scale I never dreamt possible.

In the leaflet we described the symptoms as they had been

reported to us: 'like shards of glass in the baby's mouth', 'shark's teeth'. These were unusual descriptions, but have been repeated time and again by mothers desperate to find a solution to the pain of breastfeeding and healthcare professionals who have run out of solutions.

Within three years it seemed that the majority of babies had symptoms of thrush and their mothers were being prescribed treatment in the first few weeks – sometimes in the first few days – after delivery. The one thing that we had focused on when writing the leaflet was that the mothers we had encountered had *previously had pain-free feeding and that this pain came on after feeds*. The mothers I was hearing from later were describing agonising breastfeeds, but they had never been pain-free. In addition they described pain worse in one breast, or only in one breast. This did not fit with our research and we wondered what had happened.

I began to question mothers from an opposite viewpoint, assuming that they didn't have thrush until every other possibility had been excluded. This was different from other healthcare professionals, who seemed to be treating for thrush 'just in case'. The problem was that having started on a medical pathway, it was hard to stop. If it wasn't thrush, there were circulatory problems suggesting Raynaud's phenomenon (see page 96–98). It was (and still is) very difficult to persuade mothers who had been treated for thrush but who still had symptoms that we needed to go back to basics. They often wanted to treat with other drugs or stronger doses, sometimes for weeks at a time. They subjected their healthcare professionals to extreme pressure to prescribe and would contact me for support in this campaign.

My first question was and still is – are the symptoms in both breasts equally after every feed? Thrush is very contagious. Transfer from one breast to the other via the baby's mouth is inevitable. If either mother or baby contracts it, then transfer to the other is also inevitable, which is why both need treatment. Pain that varies between the two breasts suggests that attachment is much more likely to be the cause. If the pain is worse in the mornings it is likely that the milk ducts have become over-full overnight, perhaps because of less frequent feedings or ineffective drainage. If the pain doesn't occur after every feed that excludes thrush too.

My second question is whether there is any change in the shape or colour of the nipple after feeds and specifically whether the tip of the nipple goes white after feeds. This is also strongly suggestive of less than perfect attachment, as is the response that breastfeeding is particularly painful on latching and during the feed. Many mothers have been told that their latch is perfect and thus assume that their pain must have another cause; sadly, they have been let down by their supporters. No latch is 'perfect' if it is causing the mother pain!

Raynaud's phenomenon

Raynaud's is a condition associated with poor circulation to the extremities – fingers, toes, noses, ear lobes, nipples and the penis. It can also be linked to severe migraines and with autoimmune conditions such as scleroderma, rheumatoid arthritis, Sjögren's syndrome and lupus. Around 1 in 10 people with Raynaud's go on to develop an autoimmune condition.

Sadly this seems to be another scapegoat for sore nipples. I have come across mothers who describe white nipples after breastfeeds and have been advised to ask their GP to prescribe nifedipine to treat them. This is a drug that passes into breastmilk at low levels and is therefore safe to be taken by the breastfeeding mother, but it is not without side-effects. It tends to cause violent headaches and hot flushes, which are uncomfortable and mean that not everyone can tolerate it.

Let us take a step back and look at the symptoms of Raynaud's. Symptoms were captured by a mother on her camera phone and published in the *BMJ* (Holmen, 2009). They showed a rapid change from white to purple and then red. This is very different to noting a white nipple after a feed, which could be explained by compression of the nipple between the baby's tongue and roof of the mouth. This pressure cuts off the blood supply, leading to a white nipple immediately after the feed, which can be accompanied by pain as the blood flows back into the area. In this case nifedipine, which acts by opening up blood vessels, will not help symptoms. So suggesting that the drug is prescribed to see if it might help is unethical for four reasons:

- It has medicalised a breastfeeding issue
- It has missed an opportunity to optimise attachment
- It has exposed mother and baby to an unnecessary drug
- The much-maligned GP has been asked to prescribe an unlicensed drug unnecessarily

Mothers with Raynaud's will have a history of poor circulation, a close relative with symptoms or an auto-immune condition. In the absence of these, the chances are low of there being circulatory problems in the nipples during breastfeeding. My diagnostic criteria is to ask the mother whether she automatically covers and rubs her nipples after a feed (to restore blood flow), and if the pain comes on when she gets cold, for example when walking down the freezer aisle in the supermarket.

It is important to treat or at least recognise that Raynaud's phenomenon can affect breastfeeding and cause pain. Not all mothers want to take medication and may find that heat applied to the nipples after feeds (e.g. a warm wheat bag or warmed oil) or sheepskin breast pads may be sufficient. Medication matters, but not when the answer may be more simple and basic.

	Total duration of breastfeeding					
	0%	<2w	2-6w	6w-4m	4-6m	>6m
Engorgement	36	20	28	33	45	46
Worry about having enough milk	35	29	40	44	43	32
Baby having difficulty taking the breast/not sucking effectively	21	31	30	24	19	14
Blocked milk ducts	14	4	10	12	15	18
Mastitis	12	5	11	11	16	15
Thrush	5	2	7	10	7	9
Tongue-tie	8	4	6	5	4	5
Abscess	1	1	1	2	2	1

Reasons mothers gave for stopping breastfeeding with age (McAndrew, 2012)

Not enough milk

Concerns about not having enough milk are common at all ages and durations of breastfeeding, as in the data above taken from the Infant Feeding Survey 2010. Why? To me it seems to stem from a lack of confidence in our bodies to nurture our babies. So often books, and sometimes health professionals, talk about the volume of milk to be consumed at a feed. We can't measure the volume of breastmilk. Some babies are very efficient feeders and can access all they need in 5-10 minutes, others take 20 minutes or longer. The mothers at either end of this spectrum can be concerned they don't have enough milk. It is a common misconception that the longer the baby spends at the breast, the more milk they consume. Babies can spend a long time appearing to suckle but doing little more than mouthing the nipple. This may be comfort sucking, and is not a problem, but it should not be mistaken for nutritive sucking achieving significant milk transfer.

Mothers who feel that they don't have enough milk may decide to add bottles of formula to supplement their milk supply, while others decide to give up breastfeeding altogether. However, some women look to medication to increase their supply. The first call is often fenugreek, a herb purported to increase milk supply and widely recommended on breastfeeding forums.

In a study in Western Australia of 304 questionnaires from breastfeeding women, 24.3% reported the use of at least one herb to increase breastmilk supply. The most commonly used herbs were fenugreek (18.4%), ginger (11.8%), dong quai (7.9%), chamomile (7.2%), garlic (6.6%) and blessed thistle (5.9%). Only 28.6% of users notified their doctor of their decision to use herbal medicine(s) during breastfeeding; 71.6% had previously refused or avoided conventional medicine treatments due to concerns about the safety of their breastfed infants. What concerns me is that 43.4% perceived herbal medicines to be safer than conventional medicines (Sim, 2013).

Research to confirm the efficacy of herbal galactagogues (milk-producing preparations) is lacking. There are many anecdotal reports about the effectiveness of fenugreek. A survey conducted by La Leche League in 2004 reported positive effects in milk supply in approximately 75% of lactating women (Renfree, 2004). According to the Academy of Breastfeeding Medicine (2011), most studies are of small samples and lack consistent protocols. The ABM goes on to comment 'herbs mentioned as galactagogues include fenugreek, goat's rue, milk thistle (silybum marianum), oats, dandelion, millet, seaweed, anise, basil, blessed thistle, fennel seeds, marshmallow, and many others.' Although beer is used in some cultures, alcohol may actually reduce milk production. A barley component of beer (even non-alcoholic beer) can increase prolactin secretion, but there are 'no systematic studies' and 'there is no hard evidence for causal effect'. The mechanism(s) of action for most herbals are unknown. Most of them have not been scientifically evaluated, but traditional use suggests safety and possible efficacy.

Whether fenugreek transfers into milk is unknown. However, untoward effects have only rarely been reported. Hypoglycaemia (lowering of blood sugars) has been noted in doses over 25g per day (levels normally used to increase milk supply are 1–6g), and it has been reported to increase the anticoagulant effect of warfarin. There is also one report of suspected gastrointestinal bleeding in a premature infant. Fenugreek is listed in the US as a GRAS herbal (Generally Regarded As Safe). A maple syrup odour in urine, faeces and sweat is commonly noted.

Fenugreek, therefore, has an unsubstantiated effect on increasing milk supply and appears relatively safe. However, we know that breastmilk supply is increased by frequent, effective breastfeeding (or expressing). So do we need herbs as well, or just more confidence in our bodies? In cultures where breastfeeding is normal and widespread, concerns about having enough milk are far rarer than in our own society. In my view better breastfeeding support would reduce mothers' reliance on herbal preparations.

Colic

A baby with colic can be very difficult to cope with. Colic is often defined as 'spasmodic contraction of smooth muscle causing pain and discomfort for at least three hours a day on more than three days a week for at least three weeks' (Wessel, 1954). Was Wessel ever the father of a baby with colic? His description doesn't acknowledge the agony that the parents perceive that the baby is experiencing and the distress that it causes.

I used to get many questions about the treatment of colic, but these seem to have been replaced by questions about reflux or silent reflux, or cows' milk protein intolerance (see below).

So far, no one has been able to explain why some babies have colic. It classically appears during the evening and parents spend hours walking up and down the room, massaging the tummy, rocking, giving colic drops and sometimes crying as much as the baby. The babies scream and draw their knees up to their chests, which suggests tummy pain, but this is in fact the only way they have of showing distress.

In most cases symptoms resolve between three and five months of age. The incidence is reported to be around 25% of all babies and is more common in formula-fed babies (Balon, 1997). It is twice as common in babies of mothers who smoke.

The evidence-base for medication to treat colic is poor. Simethicone drops are probably the most widely used (Infacol, Dentinox). The ingredient is purported to bind the bubbles of wind together so they are more easily passed. One piece of research (Metcalf, 1994) studied 83 babies aged 2–8 weeks, treating them with either simethicone drops or placebo and then swapping the treatments over. The results are shown in the table overleaf.

Drug	Positive Response %
Simethicone	28
Placebo	27
Simethicone and Placebo	20

Results of study comparing simethicone drops with placebo (Metcalf, 1994)

The results of the study, which lasted 3 to 10 days in each treatment period, were not statistically significant. The authors concluded that simethicone was no more effective than placebo, although it may be perceived as so by desperate parents who feel that at least they have done something.

Other interventions studied, including early response to symptoms (not leaving the baby to cry), or reducing stimulation (keeping baby in a dark, quiet room), have also failed to show evidence of benefit (Lucassen, 1998).

In 2000 the journal *Bandolier* reported that there were no evidence-based treatments for colic, but that babies do grow out of it.

Treatment	Number of Trials	Number of infants in studies	Comment
Simethicone	3	272	Three trials with adequate double blinding showed no evidence of efficacy

Dicyclomine	3	134	Dicyclomine better than placebo in three trials. Serious, adverse effects on infants reported. Drug contraindicated in infants less than 6 months of age
Soy Formula	2	158	One study showed good improvement, analysis not possible in larger second study
Increased Carrying	2	94	No effect
Hypoallergenic formula	2	72	Indication that hypoallergenic formula has a beneficial effect in two studies
Sucrose	2	72	Sucrose appears to be briefly effective
Lactase Enzymes	2	44	No benefit over placebo
Hypoallergenic diet	1	115	Breastfed and bottle-fed infants included. May be a reduction of daily colic symptoms of 25%, but complicated design and inconsistent result reporting

Herbal Tea	1	68	Small effect in single study, but no nutritional value and inappropriate in small babies
Fibre-enriched formula	1	54	No effect
Decreased Stimulation	1	42	Bare significance in trial with potential for bias
Dairy elimination diet	1	40	No benefit
Car ride simulator	1	32	No effect
Parent Training	1	14	No effect in tiny flawed trial

Summary of trials of interventions for colic (Bandolier, 2000)

However, in 2004 Bandolier looked again at the evidence on lactase drops (Colief). There was limited evidence of effectiveness when the milk was pre-incubated. Kanabar (2001) studied 53 babies. The lactase drops were either:

- Added to formula milk and left refrigerated for four hours before warming to feed to the baby
- Added to a small amount of expressed breastmilk which was then given to the baby at the end of the feed

Kanabar noted that crying time was reduced in all babies, but reached statistical significance in the 32 families who were compliant with the protocol. The remainder did not respond to the same extent.

The Colief website instructs parents of breastfed babies to:

> 'Express a few tablespoons of breast milk into a sterilised container. Add four drops of Colief and feed it back to the baby using a sterilised plastic spoon. Immediately start breastfeeding as normal... If drops were given directly to the baby, the acid in the upper digestive tract would quickly change the nature of the enzyme and render Colief ineffective. However, mixing four drops of Colief with a little expressed foremilk appears to protect the active ingredient, lactase enzyme. The foremilk preparation provides a lining to the baby's upper digestive tract, mixing with the breast milk and working to reduce the lactose level of the milk.
>
> We believe that in this form, the enzyme has an effective 'working life' of approximately 30 minutes. Laboratory trials have shown that four drops of Colief in 3.38 fl oz of infant milk at body temperature will break down approximately 70% of the lactose in 30 minutes.'

The evidence quoted to support the use of Colief is that:

> 'Colief was tested at Cork University Hospital, Ireland, by Professor Kearney in the early 1990s to demonstrate that a lactose-reduced feed was effective in reducing infant colic. His results were presented to the Royal College of Paediatricians at its annual meeting in spring

1994 and published in the Journal of Human Nutrition and Dietetics in September 1998. These results were confirmed in a larger study recently completed at Guy's Hospital, London, by Dr Dipak Kanabar and published in the Journal of Human Nutrition and Dietetics in October 2001.'

What this shows is that a product costing £9.99 for 15ml (August 2016) relies on the evidence of testing just 53 babies. The manufacturer's instructions do not include pre-incubation, which the trial found was essential to efficacy. To me this isn't good evidence-based practice, and yet this drug is prescribable on the NHS.

The clinical knowledge summary for GPs, supported by NICE 2014, suggests that the following information is given to parents with a baby suffering from colic:

- Reassure the parents that their baby is well, they are not doing something wrong, the baby is not rejecting them, and that colic is a common phase that will pass within a few months.
- Holding the baby through the crying episode may be helpful. However, if there are times when the crying feels intolerable, it is best to put the baby down somewhere safe (such as their cot) and take a few minutes' 'time out'.

Other strategies that may help to soothe a crying infant include:

- Gentle motion (for example pushing the pram or rocking the crib).
- 'White noise' (for example from a vacuum cleaner, hairdryer, or running water).
- Bathing the baby in a warm bath.

- Encourage parents to look after their own well-being by:
- Asking family and friends for support — parents need to be able to take a break.
- Resting when the baby is asleep.
- Meeting other parents with babies of the same age.

Lactose intolerance

Lactose intolerance is often blamed for colic, on the premise that excess lactose passing undigested into the lower gut becomes a substrate for bifidobacteria and lactobacilli, producing lactic acid and hydrogen. The rapid production of hydrogen distends the gut, causing pain. Meanwhile the osmotic pressure sucks in water to the gut, producing acidic diarrhoea.

However, primary lactose intolerance (an inherited condition) is rare and shows itself within a few days of birth. It is characterised by severe diarrhoea, vomiting and dehydration, as well as failure to thrive.

Savilahti et al (1983) identified only 16 cases of congenital lactase deficiency over 17 years, despite the fact that the genes are very common in Finland. In each case the mother reported watery diarrhoea, usually after the first breastfeed but up to 10 days after birth. Poor absorption of lactose was confirmed between 3 and 90 days after delivery, at which time all infants were dehydrated and 15 of the 16 weighed less than at birth. On a lactose-free diet the children all caught up with their growth.

Secondary lactose intolerance is common in some premature babies: only 40% of babies born at 35 weeks have significant lactase and few born at 28 weeks have any. It can also occur after a gut infection, due to damage to the villae in the gut. Exposure of the baby to antibiotics via the mother's breastmilk can produce similar symptoms, but these resolve with continued breastfeeding. Lactose intolerance is common in adults, as our production of lactase naturally declines after the age of two. A transitory lactase deficiency is simply too much lactose for the lactase available at that moment in time.

In 1988 Woolridge and Fisher identified that an imbalance in milk transfer could occur when the baby had less than perfect attachment to the breast. The rapid transit time of lactose-rich milk produces symptoms of loose bowel motions which may be green and frothy, together with excess wind and tummy discomfort in the baby. The solution is help to improve attachment and drainage of the breast at every feed.

There is also much confusion between lactose intolerance and cows' milk protein intolerance. Lactose is the sugar in all mammalian milks. The level is independent of the mother's consumption and hardly varies (some mothers try unnecessarily to avoid lactose, which is a filler in many tablets). The level of lactase (the enzyme required to breakdown the sugar) does vary and low levels may result in symptoms of excess lactose.

Cows' milk protein allergy/intolerance comes from a reaction to the protein in dairy products. The level in breastmilk can be influenced by the consumption of foods and drinks by the mother. (See below).

Reflux

Some reflux (gastro-oesophageal reflux) occurs in most babies. In other words babies spit up, or 'posset', regurgitating small amounts of curdled milk. In a paper in 2004 Craig said that 40–50% of babies under the age of three months bring up their feeds spontaneously at least once a day. Does this mean that they need medication? Not as frequently as it is prescribed or recommended. Regurgitation declines over the first six months and dramatically after 12 months (NICE 2015). This corresponds with babies learning to sit and stand.

Age	Percentage
0–3 m	50
4 m	67
6 m	61
7 m	21
12 m	5

Regurgitation of at least 1 episode a day with age (Nelson, 1997)

It seems that mothers have become increasingly worried by spit up/posseting/vomiting, when in fact this is normal behaviour. Does it have anything to do with the marketing of specialised formulas that claim to help the milk 'stay down'? These formulas are thickened with corn, rice or maize starch and the evidence to support their effectiveness is often lacking. See First Steps Nutrition Trust's report on specialised infant milks (available free online) for more information. It is important to note that the manufacturer guidelines on how to make up thickened infant milks are not in line with current recommendations for making up infant formula safely, since they suggest using cold or hand-hot water rather than water boiled and left to cool to 70 degrees C. This is because anti-reflux milk made up with water at 70 degrees C is likely to become lumpy. However, if the milk is made up with cold or hand-hot water, there is an increased risk of bacteria being present in the milk. Some thickened milks are also associated with constipation.

According to NICE (2015), we should investigate or prescribe for babies with reflux if an infant or child without overt regurgitation presents with more than one of the following: unexplained feeding difficulties, distressed behaviour, faltering growth, chronic cough, hoarseness, or a single episode of pneumonia.

Most cases of reflux clear up without intervention, but simple changes can help reduce symptoms.

- Feed more frequently and respond at the baby's first cues that he/she is hungry – crying is a late sign of hunger and will increase the air swallowed, making regurgitation of feeds more likely.
- Keep the baby upright after feeds over your shoulder ideally for at least 30 minutes. Do not put the baby down in a car seat where he or she may become somewhat slumped. Try not to jiggle or move the baby too much as the feed settles.
- Take time to burp the baby in a sitting position with his/her head supported with your hand – be prepared with a muslin cloth over your shoulder and a bib on the baby to protect clothing (and reduce washing!)
- Put the baby to sleep flat on his or her back. You can raise the whole of the top of the crib, for example, by putting books underneath the legs, but do not use pillows to raise the baby's head.
- Seek support with breastfeeding to ensure the baby has access to all the milk and that the breasts are well drained.

Caring for a baby with reflux is difficult, exhausting and confusing. It may be isolating as the mother may be concerned about the baby posseting when she is out. The mother may feel a loss of confidence as well as exhaustion. Being told that her baby's symptoms are normal may be reassuring, but may also leave her feeling helpless.

In most cases the first treatment prescribed for reflux is alginate (Gaviscon Infant sachets). The sachets are prepared by mixing the contents with 5ml (1 teaspoon) of cooled boiled water until a smooth paste is formed, then another 10ml (2 teaspoons) of cooled boiled water is added. The solution is given part way through each feed using a spoon, syringe or feeding bottle. Expressed breastmilk may be substituted for the boiled water. This is not an easy process as it should be made up freshly. A baby used to being breastfed as soon as he/she stirs has to wait for the Gaviscon to be prepared, assuming mum has her expressed milk ready. In addition, alginate is also associated with constipation and babies may become increasingly distressed. Anecdotally mothers find it a hard medication to administer, and may abandon it and/or breastfeeding in frustration. The recommended trial period is one to two weeks, and if it hasn't helped it should be stopped.

Many more babies (and mothers!) find better relief with ranitidine. NICE 2015 suggests that acid-suppressing drugs, such as proton pump inhibitors (PPIs e.g. ranitidine) or H2 receptor antagonists (H2RAs e.g. omeprazole), should not be used to treat overt regurgitation in infants and children occurring as isolated symptoms. However, they can be used if the growth is faltering or the baby is showing signs of distress after feeds. Some ranitidine solutions contain large amounts of alcohol as a preservative and babies may refuse this. Discussion with the pharmacist may help mothers locate a product with less or no alcohol.

Reflux is not the same as Gastro-Oesophageal Reflux Disease (GORD), in which the baby does not gain weight and vomits frequently and forcefully. Salvatore (2002) reported that in up to half the cases of GORD in infants younger than one year, there may be an association with cows' milk protein allergy/intolerance (see below). Heine (2006) noted that infants with these conditions often respond to hypoallergenic formula or a maternal elimination diet, but only a few randomised clinical trials have been conducted.

Cows' milk protein allergy/intolerance

Cows' milk protein allergy (CMPA) is being diagnosed with increasing frequency. It can affect people of all ages but is most prevalent in infants. It affects between 2 and 7.5% of formula-fed babies and 0.5% of exclusively breastfed babies. Exclusively breastfed babies develop CMPA as a result of milk proteins from products the mother has eaten transferring through breastmilk. The level of cows' milk protein present in breast milk is 100,000 times lower than that in cows' milk. Most reactions to cows' milk protein in exclusively breastfed babies are mild or moderate, and severe forms of CMPA are very rare. It is thought that immunomodulators present in breastmilk and differences in the gut flora of breastfed and formula-fed infants may contribute to this (Ludman, 2013).

Secretory immunoglobulin A (sIgA) in breastmilk 'paints' a protective coating on the inside of a baby's intestines to prevent penetration by potential allergens such as foreign proteins. In the first few days after birth the gut is particularly permeable to foreign proteins, which is why it is particularly important to avoid giving babies formula in the first few days.

However, according to data from the Infant Feeding Survey 2010, 31% of babies received additional feeds before they left hospital – formula, water or glucose. This was heavily associated with being premature, in special care units or receiving treatment for jaundice. Nevertheless 14% of mothers were advised to give other fluids and 10% of mothers chose to do so while still in hospital. It is interesting to note that giving fluids other than breastmilk while in hospital is associated with an increased likelihood of stopping breastfeeding in the early weeks. Is this a sign of problems not being sorted out at the beginning of the breastfeeding journey or mothers' confidence being undermined?

So of the 82% of babies who are put to the breast initially, 31% are given other fluids within the first 24 hours. Just over 57% of babies are exclusively breastfed after 24 hours. We also know that at 8–10 months 89% of mothers had given some formula in the past seven days, and for 73% of babies this was their sole source of milk. At six months just 1% of babies are exclusively breastfed. The vast majority of babies are now exposed to the cows' milk proteins in formula milk during the first six months of life while the gut is maturing.

The symptoms of cows' milk protein allergy/intolerance are many and varied as seen in the table overleaf.

Why Mothers' Medication Matters

Organ Involvement	Symptoms
Gastrointestinal Tract	· Frequent Regurgitation · Vomiting or Diarrhoea · Constipation (with/without perineal rash) · Blood in Stool · Iron Deficiency Anaemia
Skin	· Atopic Dermatitis · Swelling of lips or eye lids (angio-oedema) · Urticaria unrelated to acute infections, drug intake or other causes
Respiratory Tract	· Runny nose, otitis media
(unrelated to infection)	· Chronic cough or wheezing
General	· Persistent distress or colic (wailing/irritable for ≥3 h per day) at least 3 days/week over a period of >3 weeks

Symptoms of cows' milk protein allergy (developed from VandenPlas, 2007)

The reaction may be mediated by IgE (anaphylaxis, urticaria) if it occurs immediately following consumption of cows' milk protein, or non IgE (GI reactions, eczema, GOR), which may occur several hours or even days after consumption. The immune system responds to the protein casein or the whey found in cows' milk (NICE 2011).

Where CMPA is suspected in a breastfed baby, the recommended treatment is for the mother to remove all sources of products containing cows' milk from her diet, ideally under medical supervision. Mothers should be prescribed a supplement of 1000mg of calcium and 10 mcg of vitamin D (two tablets) every day. It will usually take between two and four weeks for symptoms in the baby to disappear. It is suggested that milk is then reintroduced to ensure that this has been the cause of the symptoms (Ludman et al 2013, NICE 2011), but many mothers will be reluctant to do this. Care should also be taken with the weaning diet and appropriate alternative sources of calcium included under dietetic supervision. There is generally no need to add special prescription formula for weaning if breastfeeding continues.

A diagnosis of cows' milk protein allergy has many ramifications for mother and baby. A mother should not be asked to remove products containing cows' milk protein lightly, as it is not straightforward and may compromise her nutritional status without dietetic support. She should be offered referral to a breastfeeding expert to address issues around optimal attachment.

There is a lot of technical information in this section and you may be feeling confused. Why have I got into this level of detail? Firstly, it's because I so often see mothers on social media being told that their babies have CMPA, for a variety of reasons ranging from reflux to colic to rashes to sleeping and behaviour, all of which could be within the norm for a breastfed baby. No two babies are the same. Every one of us is an individual and we don't have to conform to a pattern of 'perfection'. I hope that this section is both reassuring and helpful.

If a baby has obvious signs of allergy, with severe vomiting or blood in the stools, clearly this needs to be investigated, and it makes sense to try reducing dairy in the mother's diet. Some people notice an immediate difference. For others it takes several weeks. To remove all dairy is a major commitment as it is hidden in many foods. It isn't as simple as avoiding butter, cheese and milk. It means asking about the ingredients in restaurant meals and avoiding most convenience foods, including cakes, biscuits, chocolate and ice cream.

If the baby's symptoms improve when the mother removes dairy from her diet, there is no reason to consider specialised formula as long as the mother is willing to continue to breastfeed on this restricted diet. I have come across many scenarios where there have been recommendations to GPs from dieticians to prescribe the hydrolysed formula 'just in case'. I have even heard of consultations with dieticians where there was a stack of formula waiting to be taken home, regardless of what the mother thought. At a cost of around £30 a tin this can significantly affect the prescribing budget locally. Mothers may see specialised formula as a magic wand to fix problems – it isn't. I have had mothers ask me about relactation (restarting breastfeeding) when they regret having stopped in order to switch to the formula, or have been told that they can't breastfeed for four weeks until their milk has been cleared of allergens, while their babies are fed hydrolysed formula milk. There is certainly a need for specialised formula, but in many cases the breastfeeding relationship can be preserved, and the mother can decide for herself what to do if she is given good breastfeeding support and accurate, independent, evidence-based information.

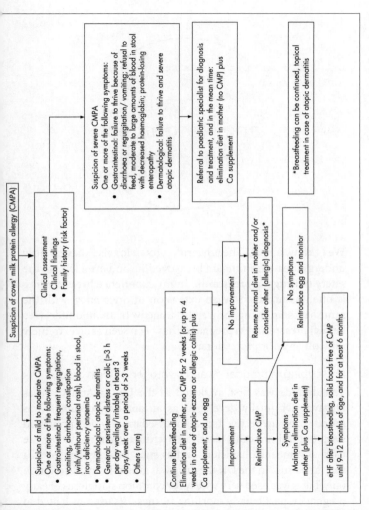

Algorithm for the diagnosis and management of cows' milk protein allergy (CMPA) in exclusively breastfed infants. (VandenPlas, 2007)

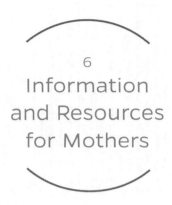

6

Information and Resources for Mothers

We know that healthcare professionals have little undergraduate training on breastfeeding and even less on the safety of drugs in breastmilk. In my experience breastfeeding is often assumed to be an extension of pregnancy, with the same risks applying. Since the tragedy of thalidomide (see below) prescribing in pregnancy has been seen as an extremely difficult area for professionals.

Prescribing in pregnancy and teratogenic (birth defect) risk

Thalidomide was first marketed in the UK in April 1958 as Distaval. Originally developed as an anti-convulsant, it was found to be ineffective but a good sedative, which promoted sleep but did not cause death in overdose (many sedatives are used as a means of suicide) and as such was highlighted as a very safe drug. In the UK the drug was available on prescription only, but it was used very widely for common symptoms of early pregnancy, particularly morning sickness. Its use was halted in November 1961, but deformed babies continued to be born because of the use of drugs already in homes and medicine cupboards. To produce teratogenic defects it had to have been taken when the embryo was most sensitive, 34 to 50 days after the beginning of the mother's last period.

Thalidomide is associated predominantly with limb defects and these were certainly the most common. However, almost any organ of the body could be affected. The second largest number of abnormalities involved the ears, the eyes, the nerve supplies to the face, the eye muscles and the tear glands. Internally the heart, kidneys and urinary tract, the gut and the genital tract could all be affected. The early death rate (before the first birthday) among babies exposed to thalidomide in the womb was about 40%, largely as a result of serious internal malformations, which is why the limb abnormalities became most associated with the drug. About 10,000 babies were affected worldwide.

These tragic births made everyone very aware of the consequences of taking medication in the early weeks of pregnancy when the embryo is developing the major organs. The treatment of common acute illnesses in early pregnancy is complicated. The period of greatest risk is between the first and eighth week of pregnancy. With chronic ongoing conditions the mother may seek pre-conception advice about whether to stop her medication, change it, take a higher dose of folic acid or consider the risks of continuing. No drugs have been tested in clinical trials in humans to ascertain whether they will cause abnormalities – it would be unethical to do so. It would also be impossible to recruit enough people to ensure that rare abnormalities were captured by the research. The data we have is retrospectively collected, largely by the completion of 'yellow cards'. Drugs may be tested on animals, but the results are not always transferable to humans.

So far only 30 drugs have been shown to cause major abnormalities, according to the Motherisk team in Toronto (Pole,

2000). In a study looking at the teratogenic risk of drugs used to treat nausea and vomiting in pregnancy, the drugs were labelled according to safety and the participants were asked to rank them. Even health professionals reading the labels describing safe drugs rated them as unsafe and, despite evidence-based information, were reluctant to change that view. Words such as 'malformation' and 'abnormality' increased concerns even though the information provided was essentially the same for all drugs.

All pregnancies have a background risk of foetal abnormalities of around 2–3%. In many cases if the embryo is badly affected the body will naturally miscarry, particularly if the exposure was in the first 14 days after conception (the pre-embryonic period). Many of us worry about what we did between the date of our last period, conception and finding out we are pregnant. What about that bottle of wine? What about the painkillers for that headache? In the vast majority of cases all will be well and it seems as if the body naturally knows how to protect and produce a perfectly formed baby. Of course this doesn't mean we should take unnecessary risks, nor that taking folic acid isn't vitally important.

The foetus is most at risk from teratogens in weeks three to eight after conception (the embryonic period) when the major organs are developing. For example, exposure to sodium valproate during this time may result in spina bifida, as the neural tube closes between day 17 and day 30 after conception. Cleft palate is most likely to develop around 36 days after conception.

Week nine up until birth is termed the foetal period and babies are less susceptible to damage, although some structures continue to form. During this period there is more likely to be a reduction in growth or within organs: for example, warfarin may cause bleeding in the brain, while ibuprofen and other non-steroidal anti-inflammatory drugs can cause premature closure of the ductus arteriosus, producing neonatal pulmonary hypertension.

Fluoxetine can produce severe drowsiness after birth.

Teratogens can also prevent implantation, cause abortion, produce intrauterine growth retardation or cause foetal death (Lee, 2000). Drugs should be avoided in pregnancy unless they are essential. However this sentence can cause anxiety in many women who need to take medication for chronic conditions, so discussion of the risks should ideally take place in the period *before* conception. With some drugs higher doses of folic acid (5mg daily) are recommended. It may be possible to reduce the number of drugs a mother is taking, or discontinue drugs temporarily (e.g. statins). Realistically a discussion of the relative risk of the increase of teratogenicity compared with the risk to the mother's health should be held, allowing the (prospective) parents to make an informed choice.

Drugs most likely to cause teratogenic abnormalities in the baby

Only a few drugs are proven teratogens. The most commonly prescribed are shown in the table below. However, because it is impossible to design studies large enough to identify risk on an epidemiological basis, no drug has been proven to be safe in pregnancy.

Drug	Teratogenic Risk
ACE inhibitors e.g. enalapril, ramipril, perindopril	Angiotensin-Converting Enzyme (ACE) inhibitors are normally stopped when planning a pregnancy
Statins e.g. simvastatin, atorvastatin	Statins are teratogenic and ideally should be stopped at least three months prior to conception.

Anti-epilepsy Drugs (AEDs)	Most AEDs are teratogenic, although the risk is reduced with monotherapy (one single drug). Some AEDs are potentially less likely to cause problems, but the risk to the foetus needs to be balanced with the risk of seizures in the mother, which puts both the mother and the baby at risk of harm. Phenytoin can retard foetal growth within the uterus, cause an abnormally small head, lead to mental retardation and affect normal development of facial features. Sodium valproate carries a high risk of neural tube defects. Mothers on any AEDs should take 5mg folic acid.
Alcohol	Foetal Alcohol Syndrome is seen in babies born to mothers who drink excessive amounts of alcohol and no safe threshold amount can be defined.
Herbal Medications	There is little information on safety during pregnancy so these should be avoided.
Antibiotics	Penicillins, erythromycin and cephalosporins are safe. Trimethoprim interferes with folate metabolism and so should be avoided in the first trimester. Tetracycline can cause a yellow staining of the teeth and reduce growth of long bones. Aminoglycosides such as gentamycin cause deafness.

Warfarin	Causes foetal warfarin syndrome.
Lithium	Where possible lithium should be avoided in pregnancy, especially in the first trimester, as it can sometimes cause an abnormality of the heart valves. All women on lithium should have a high resolution ultrasound scan and foetal echocardiography at 18–20 weeks of pregnancy.
Cocaine	Causes cardiovascular and central nervous system defects.

Foetal abnormalities due to exposure to drugs in pregnancy (after Lee, 2000)

Frequently it seems that prescribing decisions and recommendations about medication for breastfeeding mothers are similar to those in pregnancy. This means a cautious approach, and this, in my experience, often means mothers are told that they cannot take medicines while they are breastfeeding. However, breastfeeding is not the same as pregnancy, as we have seen.

So what can you do if you need medical help and are not ready to stop or even interrupt breastfeeding? None of us is in a good place to pick an argument when we feel poorly, and it can be helpful to be armed with information.

An important tool to use in discussions with any medical practitioner, be that a doctor, pharmacist, nurse, podiatrist, anaesthetist, dentist, physiotherapist, optician or any of the others you may consult is the NICE guideline on prescribing, quoted in Chapter 1.

Where to find evidence

Why might you be advised to stop or interrupt breastfeeding, and how can you challenge this? It could be that the *British National Formulary* (*BNF*) does not provide sufficient information for an informed decision (as we have already discussed). It could be that during his/her training your medical professional (doctor, pharmacist, nurse, consultant, anaesthetist, podiatrist) has been told that prescribing outside of the medical licence is risky and shouldn't be undertaken. Actually we use many drugs outside of their licence (off-label) regularly. For example, gabapentin, which is a drug used to treat epilepsy, is routinely used to help with neuropathic pain. Hospital consultants often use drugs in an unorthodox way based on their clinical experience, for example using drugs to treat children which are not licensed for those under 12. These clinical decisions are made using a thoughtful, experienced decision-making process after consultation with the patient or their parent/guardian. In general practice healthcare professionals need to prescribe for a wide variety of conditions based on a general understanding. The safety of drugs in breastmilk should be seen as a speciality and expert sources consulted.

What are these expert sources? There is one free online database which provides research-based, up-to-date information on the safety of many, if not all, drugs in breastmilk. The database is called LactMed (toxnet.nlm.nih.gov/cgi-bin/sis/htmlgen?LACTMED). It includes information under several headings:

- Summary
- Measured drug levels from available studies which are referenced
- Effects in breastfed infants from the same studies

- Effects on lactation and breastmilk
- Alternative drugs to consider (with HTML links to those alternatives)
- References

It is possible to search LactMed using the generic (chemical name) or the brand name of a drug. It is a database compiled in the USA, so some names are spelt differently and some drugs will not appear as they are not used in America (for example paracetamol is acetaminophen; midazolam is known as Versed). In some countries, such as Eire and the USA, drugs are much more likely to be known by their trade (branded names), while in England we tend to use generic names that cover several brands.

LactMed is freely available for mothers and healthcare professionals to search and was recommended by NICE PH11.

There are a couple of useful books that you could recommend to your healthcare professionals. *Medications and Mother's Milk* is by Tom Hale, an American clinical pharmacologist who has also established the InfantRisk Centre (www.infantrisk.com), which takes queries from healthcare professionals and mothers as well as promoting research and education pertaining to medication safety for pregnant and breastfeeding mothers.

My own book *Breastfeeding and Medication* was published by Routledge in 2013. My aim was to answer all the questions healthcare professionals might have.

The UK Medicines Information Service (UKMI) has a specialist centre for questions relating to the safety of drugs in breastmilk. The information has recently been included in a database provided by the Specialist Pharmacy Service (www.sps.nhs.uk/?s=drugs+in+lactation).

UKMI takes telephone calls from healthcare professionals

and there is an online enquiry form. This is the official, NHS-funded information centre for queries relating to the safety of drugs in breastmilk.

I have written over 50 fact sheets on common conditions for the Breastfeeding Network (www.breastfeedingnetwork. org.uk/drugs-factsheets/). These have all been written using evidence-based sources and my 20 years of experience providing information on the safety of drugs in breastmilk. The list continues to grow as new topics are raised. In the future there will be two forms of each sheet – one with general information for mothers, and another more in-depth version for healthcare professionals with full pharmacological data.

I also run a Drugs in Breastmilk Helpline for the Breastfeeding Network. You can contact me by email or on the Facebook group (www.facebook.com/ BfNDrugsinBreastmilkinformation). I am helped by a small but enthusiastic and brilliant team of administrators who signpost mothers to appropriate BfN factsheets or reassure them that I will answer as soon as possible.

So there are options to find information on the safety of drugs in breastmilk for mothers and for healthcare professionals. However, it is the use to which the information is put that is important too. Sadly some healthcare professionals dismiss any information other than that which is in the *BNF* or on their computer. They appear to perceive formula milk as equivalent to breastmilk and believe that it is easy to stop breastfeeding permanently or temporarily, and they do not give information to mothers about pumping, how to maintain lactation or how to avoid blocked ducts and mastitis. It is my great hope that we will eventually succeed in changing these attitudes.

Why is formula milk the default safe option when it comes to medication?

Why are breastmilk and formula milk seen as interchangeable? Why are we so ready to advise women to stop breastfeeding? Given all that we know about breastmilk and breastfeeding, why do some professionals not look for more information? I wish I knew. Breastfeeding should not be seen as a 'nice-to-have' lifestyle choice. It is a public health imperative. Babies who are not breastfed are at greater risk of a variety of illnesses. This has ramifications as far as their comfort is concerned – it is no fun having an ear infection, chest infection or gastric infection. For the parents there will be distress in trying to comfort a sick baby, and in a society where many mothers have to work it has implications for their employers when they take unplanned leave to care for a sick baby. There are major financial implications for the NHS too. A study of 935 babies from 13 general practices in Glasgow (McConnachie, 2004) found that breastfed babies have 15% fewer GP appointments than their formula-fed counterparts in the first six months of life, although data on duration and exclusivity of breastfeeding was not collected. According to government data the average cost of a GP appointment is £45 (2013). There were 695,233 live births in England and Wales in 2014.

In a report commissioned by Unicef UK *Preventing disease and saving resources* a multi-university academic team (Renfrew, 2012) showed that for just five illnesses, moderate increases in breastfeeding would translate into cost savings for the NHS of £40 million and tens of thousands of fewer hospital admissions and GP consultations.

Utilising a total of 25 systematic reviews and UK studies, the researchers were able to utilise robust evidence to perform economic analysis. They developed quantitative models for five outcomes:

- Four acute conditions in infants: gastrointestinal disease, respiratory disease, otitis media, and necrotising enterocolitis (NEC)
- Breast cancer in mothers.

These models found that, assuming a moderate increase in breastfeeding rates, if 45% of women exclusively breastfed for four months, and if 75% of babies in neonatal units were breastfed at discharge, every year there could be an estimated:

- 3,285 fewer hospital admissions for gastro-intestinal illness and 10,637 fewer GP consultations for this condition, with over £3.6 million saved in treatment costs annually
- 5,916 fewer lower respiratory tract infection related hospital admissions and 22,248 fewer GP consultations, with around £6.7 million saved in treatment costs annually
- 21,045 fewer acute otitis media (earache) related GP consultations, with over £750,000 saved in treatment costs annually
- 361 fewer cases of NEC, with over £6 million saved in treatment costs annually.

In total, over £17 million could be gained annually by avoiding the costs of treating just these four acute diseases in infants.

Furthermore, if half those mothers who currently do not breastfeed were to breastfeed for up to 18 months in their lifetime, for each annual cohort of around 313,000 first-time mothers there could be 865 fewer breast cancer cases, with cost savings to the health service of over £21 million, not to mention the reduction in suffering of mothers and their families.

A very modest increase in the rates of exclusive

breastfeeding could be associated with the avoidance of at least three cases of SIDS annually, averting the profound consequences for families.

While increasing breastfeeding rates to a level compatible with reducing the rates of early years obesity by as little as 5% would result in reducing annual healthcare expenditures by more than £1.6 million, sadly breastfeeding does not appear in the most recent government guidance to reduce childhood obesity.

In 2010 Jayawickrama et al carried out a study in Melbourne, Australia. They distributed an anonymous postal survey to GPs to look at their knowledge, attitudes and practices around prescribing medicines to breastfeeding mothers. They reported that doctors were concerned about the complexity of managing risk, uncertain about decision-making and needed more information, as well as being concerned for the safety of the baby. Without evidence-based information doctors admitted that they sometimes recommended cessation of breastfeeding, which they realised might be unnecessary. This largely confirmed the findings of my PhD in 2000, which looked at the experiences of 1,000 mothers, 1,000 GPs and 1,000 pharmacists in a matched area. Much of the information the GPs and pharmacists passed on to mothers was based on their own infant feeding experiences rather than evidence-based information.

Hospital admissions

In my experience a lot of queries on the safety of drugs in breastmilk arise from hospital admissions. In general or surgical wards the treatment of the mother is of paramount importance. That is right and proper, but it is also important to breastfeeding mothers that they have information on the impact of their treatment on the nursling. It seems that a variety of healthcare professionals on non-paediatric wards fail to understand this.

The questions which frequently come up are:

- Is it true I can't breastfeed for 24–48 hours after a general anaesthetic?
- I have been told that I will need strong painkillers and can't breastfeed for at least 12 hours after I stop them
- The antibiotics I have been given aren't suitable for a breastfed baby so I need to pump and dump my milk until after the course is finished and for some time after
- I have to have a scan with contrast and I am being told I can't breastfeed for 24 hours

Other points which have been raised are that breast pumps cannot be provided or borrowed from the maternity unit. In one case a mother was forbidden to use an electric pump on the ward because it would disturb the other patients, that nowhere could be provided to store expressed breastmilk, that it was taking up space and had been thrown away (without permission!), that it was a potential source of infection, that babies do not need breastmilk beyond (insert a period from 4 months) because it no longer has any goodness in it, that the mother is continuing for her own benefit, that formula milk is just as good. It is very difficult not to feel intimidated when you are being admitted to hospital. Being ill disempowers us, makes us vulnerable. Simply lying on a bed with someone leaning over you takes away your power. So it is difficult in these circumstances to argue, even when you know the information you have been given is incorrect. However, we can all try whenever we can to ask for the evidence that the healthcare professionals are using to make their recommendations.

In general wards the professionals are not expected to be experts on the safety of drugs in breastmilk, but they should be taking into account the wishes of the mother and not making personal non-evidence-based statements. The baseline in any management of a lactating mother is that medication that allows her to continue breastfeeding should be chosen if at all possible. The question should not be: 'This medication is needed, can the mother breastfeed?', but 'This mother is breastfeeding, what medication can we give her to treat her symptoms effectively while she continues to breastfeed?'

In order to make decisions professionals may need to access information from an expert source. However, above all they need to understand the importance of breastfeeding for the short and long-term health of the baby and the mother. This should never be overlooked, whatever the age of the baby.

If a mother is hospitalised, where the baby sleeps may also need consideration. If the baby is still young or, more importantly, if the mother wishes it, can the baby stay with mum on the ward? Is it possible for them to have a side room? Could another adult stay to look after the baby between feeds? Is the mother well enough to care for her baby herself, or will she need help? Is there a private area where she can breastfeed if she wants? Is a cot available or could one be brought over from the maternity unit?

If the professionals on the ward are unsure about how to care for the mother and baby, could they consult with paediatricians and staff on the maternity unit? Analgesics that are commonly used after a caesarean section are the same as those normally used post-surgery. Anaesthetics are also the same or similar.

If it is not possible for the baby to stay with the mother, is she able to pump frequently to avoid blocked ducts and mastitis? Pumping may be difficult because of the anxiety of being in hospital, worrying about the baby, who may have been left at home, and how the family is coping. All these are factors known to inhibit oxytocin and therefore the let-down reflex. Even feeling uncomfortable about a lack of privacy can make pumping difficult – a closed curtain is no guarantee that someone won't enter the cubicle. Pumping in a hospital bathroom is definitely not to be encouraged!

It may be important to note that members of staff on a general ward may be unwilling to handle the baby. So if she has had surgery, will mum be able to move freely to change the baby and move it in and out of the bassinet? I have been told that mothers have been advised that staff are not insured to touch a baby (?!), and that there may be a risk of infection. Several mothers have been told that if paediatricians are not available they cannot take any strong analgesics, in particular opiates, as there is no one to monitor the baby in the event of any adverse reaction. This seems extreme when many mothers are discharged home with these drugs.

Maintaining a supply if you need to interrupt or feel pressurised into doing so

There are occasions when you do need to interrupt breastfeeding temporarily because of medication. There are also drugs that cannot be taken during breastfeeding because of the risk to the baby and for which there is no alternative.

Sometimes we may feel that a healthcare professional has put so many doubts into our mind about the risk to the baby that we are too scared to carry on breastfeeding. One example which springs to mind is the antibiotic ciprofloxacin. This is the information from one of the product leaflets '*Ciprofloxacin is passed into human breastmilk. You must not breastfeed your child during treatment with ciprofloxacin, due to the risk of malformation of joint cartilage and other harmful effects in the breastfed infant.*' That sounds really scary doesn't it? Would you want to breastfeed your child after reading that?

The LactMed summary says:

'Fluoroquinolones such as ciprofloxacin have traditionally not been used in infants because of concern about adverse effects on the infants' developing joints. However, studies indicate little risk (Kaguelidou, 2011). The calcium in milk might decrease absorption of the small amounts of fluoroquinolones in milk (Fleiss, 1992), but insufficient data exist to prove or disprove this assertion. Use of ciprofloxacin is acceptable in nursing mothers with monitoring of the infant for possible effects on the gastrointestinal flora, such as diarrhoea or candidiasis (thrush, diaper rash). Avoiding breastfeeding for 3 to 4 hours after a dose should decrease the exposure of the infant to ciprofloxacin in breastmilk.'

Hale's *Medications and Mother's Milk* has this to say:

'Ciprofloxacin is a fluoroquinolone antibiotic primarily used for gram negative coverage and is presently the drug of choice for anthrax treatment and prophylaxis. Because it has been implicated in arthropathy in new-born animals, it is not normally used in paediatric patients. Levels secreted into breastmilk (2.26 to 3.79mg/L) are somewhat conflicting. They vary from the low to moderate range to levels that are higher than maternal serum up to 12 hours after a dose. In one study of 10 women who received 750mg every 12 hours, milk levels of ciprofloxacin ranged from 3.79 mg/L at 2 hours post-dose to 0.02 mg/L at 24 hours (Giamarellou, 1989). In another study of a single patient receiving one 500mg tablet daily at bedtime, the concentrations in maternal serum and breastmilk were 0.21µg/mL and 0.98µg/mL respectively (Gargner, 1992). Plasma levels were undetectable (<0.03 µg/mL) in the

infant. The dose to the 4 month old infant was estimated to be 0.92mg/day or 0.15mg/kg/day. No adverse effects were noted in this infant.

There has been one reported case of severe pseudomembranous colitis in an infant of a mother who self-medicated with ciprofloxacin for 6 days (Harmon, 1992). In a patient 17 days postpartum, who received 500mg orally, ciprofloxacin levels in milk were 3.02, 3.02, 3.02 and 1.98 mg/L at 4, 8, 12, and 16 hours post dose respectively (Cover, 1990). In another study of the direct application of ciprofloxacin to infants, 10 infants aged 4 days to 1 month old were given ciprofloxacin 10 to 40 mg/kg/day in 2 divided doses by slow IV infusion over 30 minutes for 10 to 20 days. Eight infants survived and 2 had greenish discoloration of the teeth at age 12-23 months. The discoloration requires further evaluation to determine the association with ciprofloxacin therapy (Lumbiganon 1991, Ghaffar 2003). If used in lactating mothers, observe the infant closely for gastrointestinal symptoms such as diarrhoea. Current studies seem to suggest that the amount of ciprofloxacin present in milk is quite low.

So when given directly to young rats, ciprofloxacin produces a type of juvenile arthritis and it is not given to children for this reason except where the benefits outweigh the risks. It is also associated with some tooth discoloration. However, the amount passing into breastmilk has not been reported to produce either of these side-effects. The *BNF* says *'amount too small to be harmful but manufacturer advises avoid'*. Despite this many mothers are advised not to take this drug and breastfeed or are too frightened to do so having read the manufacturer's leaflet. The full information is needed if we are to avoid such situations.

Ciprofloxacin should only be used for severe infections

such as urinary tract infections, which have travelled into the kidneys, when a mid-stream urine specimen has suggested that this is the drug of choice.

Pump and dump

If you do need to discard your milk for a while or, despite access to all of the information about the safety of a drug in breastmilk you decide that you do not want to expose your baby to it, you need to express (and discard) your milk with the same frequency that you would have breastfed your baby. Another example may be having a drink spiked, or in a mad moment using cocaine on a night out. Both of these cases would necessitate not breastfeeding for 48–72 hours and sadly are not that uncommon.

What you feed your baby in the meantime is your choice. Maybe you have sufficient previously expressed breastmilk in the freezer, or maybe you are going to use infant formula for the duration of your treatment. Remember that there is no difference between any of the formula milk brands, despite what the manufacturers may claim in their adverts.

Expressing breastmilk can be done by hand or by using a manual, electric or battery-operated pump. What's best for you will be a personal thing and it may take time and effort to find a method you are comfortable with. Suddenly needing to pump and dump may be a challenge. You may be able to borrow a pump from your health visitor or a friend, or you may need to buy one. One tip for expressing is to try to stay relaxed and let oxytocin help the milk let down. You do not have to turn the pump up to full power; start at a lower setting and work up to avoid hurting yourself. If you don't have a breast pump or find that you don't get on with one you can hand express your milk. Hopefully you were shown how to hand express either before or soon after birth. It is a very useful technique as you can use it anywhere, anytime you need, to relieve the symptoms of a blocked duct or mastitis or simply for comfort if your breasts are over-full. If you were not shown or did not ever try it, it may be worth a go now that you are more familiar with your breasts.

First wash your hands (although if you are going to throw the milk away this is less important, just a good habit). Have a container ready to collect the milk. Massage the breast from the outer edges of the breast towards the nipple to stimulate the let-down. You may at this stage notice that milk starts to drip. Cup your breast just behind your areola and squeeze gently, using your thumb and the rest of your fingers in a C-shape. This shouldn't hurt and you should not squeeze the nipple itself. Release the pressure, then repeat, building up a rhythm until your milk is flowing freely. When no more drops come out, move your fingers round and try a different section of your breast. Repeat on the other side. If your breasts still feel full you may want to return to the first side.

Stopping breastfeeding permanently

There are times when it is not possible to carry on breastfeeding because of medication. Examples which come to mind are lithium for bipolar disorder or chemotherapy treatment. I feel strongly that it is important that mothers have full information and are involved in the decision to stop so that they understand fully what effects the drug could potentially have on their babies. In some cases mothers find that their milk supply diminishes and even stops because of a medication. This might be furosemide, a diuretic to remove excess fluid from the body, oestrogen in the combined oral contraceptive given too soon after birth or the potential 24% reduction in milk supply caused by a single tablet of a decongestant like pseudoephedrine.

In an ideal world it is better to allow the breastmilk supply to dwindle slowly, by dropping one feed at a time or expressing/feeding only when the breasts become uncomfortably full. It may however be necessary to speed up this process, but it is still important to avoid blocked ducts and mastitis. It is possible to treat the breasts as you would in the early days of engorgement, using simple analgesics and cold savoy cabbage leaves in a firm but well-fitting bra. (Don't laugh – there are studies confirming the efficacy of cabbage leaves. They contain an enzyme which helps.) Express just enough milk to remain comfortable and frequently change breast pads, which may become soaked as milk leaks from the breasts. Restricting the fluids you are drinking will not help the milk to dry up; nor will the use of laxatives to remove water from the body.

There are two prescription drugs which have been used to dry up milk – bromocriptine and cabergoline (see pages 44–46). Bromocriptine is no longer licensed for or recommended to dry up milk as it has been linked with multiple fatalities in the USA. In Europe increased reports of rare but potentially serious or fatal side effects, particularly cardiovascular side effects (such as heart attack and stroke), neurological side effects such as seizures (fits) and psychiatric side effects (such as hallucinations and manic episodes) have contributed to concerns about use.

For the suppression of established lactation, cabergoline 0.25mg is taken every 12 hours for two days for a total of 1mg. However, this drug also has significant side effects, including headache, dizziness, fatigue or insomnia, orthostatic hypotension (feeling faint when you stand up), oedema, nose bleed, dry mouth, inhibition of lactation, nausea, constipation, anorexia and weakness. There may of course also be interactions with the drugs prescribed that have caused the cessation of breastfeeding.

What if the doctor refuses to prescribe for you if you are breastfeeding?

One mother told me that her doctor had said to her:

> *'If you insist on continuing to breastfeed there is nothing I can do to help you. You have to decide what is best for you – this fashionable fad for feeding a baby longer than six weeks or your own health. My children were all bottle fed and it never did them any harm. I don't understand what all the fuss is about.'*

It is difficult to know quite where to start in this discussion from a patient's viewpoint. It is acknowledged that patients lack confidence in a situation where the professional is seen to be in a position of power (Slowie, 1999). The mother in this case was well educated and knew that breastfeeding for six weeks was not sufficient to provide them both with the full protection which even four months of exclusive breastfeeding brings. She also knew that she was unwell and needed medication, but in itself that made her vulnerable and less able to challenge what she was being told. She left the consulting room angry, upset and disempowered. She felt that she had been insulted and treated with a lack of respect, quite apart from the lack of evidence for the statements made. She made another appointment with a different doctor the following day and was prescribed the medication she needed and continued to breastfeed. Many patients have left it there, but this mother felt that she wanted to take the matter further. She wrote to the practice manager describing what had happened, citing the evidence contradicting what the first doctor had said and suggesting that the practice should undertake some continuing professional development (CPD) on the importance of breastfeeding and the prescription of drugs to a breastfeeding mother. To her surprise she was issued with a fulsome apology and invited to meet with the practice manager to help to plan this CPD. The doctor she had encountered was a locum and in view of his attitude the practice decided not to use his services again. If you feel you can complain when you have received poor care, your feedback may help others in the future.

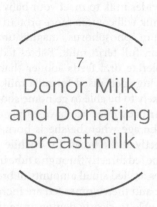

7

Donor Milk and Donating Breastmilk

The mothers of some babies born prematurely are unable or unwilling to breastfeed. In some special care baby units mothers are encouraged to express their breastmilk regardless of whether they intend to breastfeed or not, and it is seen as the most precious medicine for their babies. We know that babies who receive breastmilk when they are born prematurely have better outcomes, including lower rates of infection, better developmental outcomes and reduced stress. It is also known that breastfeeding provides analgesia during painful interventions.

Breastmilk contains high levels of immunoglobulins, which pass straight through the gaps between the milk cells in the first days after birth. These gaps close within a few days, which is one way in which drugs are prevented from passing into breastmilk, as we have already discussed.

If your baby is premature, your milk will be different from the breastmilk of a mother who gives birth at term for the first few weeks. Your body knows that your baby was born too early, and it provides milk to meet your baby's needs. For the first weeks the milk will contain more protein and fat calories, as well as calcium, phosphorus, magnesium, zinc, sodium and chloride than full-term milk. Babies fed breastmilk are often able to tolerate oral feeds sooner than they would if they were receiving specialised formula milks, which means they are more likely to be able to go home sooner. However, it may be that your baby does not have a fully developed suck, depending on the age when he/she is born, so may not be able to feed directly at the breast for a while. Your expressed breastmilk may be fed directly through a tube into the stomach. Premature babies are fed small amounts of breastmilk to help their gut mature and the volumes fed are increased gradually. Boyd et al were able to clearly demonstrate that formula-fed very low birthweight babies are at significantly increased risk of necrotising enterocolitis (NEC) compared with those fed exclusively on breastmilk (Boyd, 2007). NEC has an incidence of 2.1/1000 neonatal unit admissions, 65% of whom weigh under 1500g at birth. Sadly NEC has a risk of death of 22%, but it is significantly lower in those fed breastmilk compared with those fed on formula. This is a scenario in which breastmilk should indeed be viewed as medicine.

Expressing breastmilk over a prolonged period of time is not simple. There may be days when you are concerned about your baby's health, tired and stressed by the demands of spending hours at the unit. These factors can affect your let-down, but looking at photographs of your baby, holding a toy or a special item of clothing, or receiving a neck massage from your partner may help you relax. The volume of milk you produce depends on the number of feeds/expressing sessions that you are able to achieve. It is the frequency of expressing, rather than the time spent, which increases volume. Even if your baby is only taking small amounts it is beneficial to maximise the volume that you can produce and freeze the additional quantities (labelled in date order). Expressing during the night may seem tiring and demanding, and many new and tired mothers can be tempted to omit these. However, the level of prolactin in your body is highest in the hours of darkness, so these night feeds are vitally important.

The difficulties can begin around six weeks after birth if you are still solely expressing and unable to feed your baby directly. It can be useful to keep your baby in skin-to-skin contact as much as possible (kangaroo care). This has been shown to stabilise the baby as well as help you to feel that you have had a baby and that he doesn't belong to the special care unit! If, despite frequent expression and some stimulation from the baby near the breast, your supply begins to dip, it can be time to consider taking medication to help.

Domperidone and metoclopramide are both drugs used to treat nausea and vomiting. Both drugs are dopamine antagonists and as a side-effect can increase the level of prolactin. It is this that means they can increase milk supply (act as galactogogues). They have in the past been widely used for this purpose.

Following a European Review by the Pharmacovigilance Risk Assessment Committee (PRAC), the MHRA updated their advice on the prescription of domperidone in May 2014. They advised that domperidone is associated with a small increased risk of serious cardiac side-effects. These have been reported predominantly in over-60s with existing cardiac problems, who were taking other drugs which also cause arrhythmia, or a dose of domperidone greater than 10mg three times a day. A consensus statement by breastfeeding experts in Canada affirmed that adverse effects from domperidone given to increase lactation are exceptionally rare (www.nbci.ca/docs/Domperidone_Consensus_Statement_May_11_2012.pdf).

There are studies which confirm that these drugs effectively increase prolactin levels and breastmilk quantities with very few side-effects in mother and baby. There is a fact sheet on the Breastfeeding Network website on domperidone as a galactogogue, which has lots of information that you can share with your GP if the hospital breastfeeding team think that you would benefit and all other methods of increasing your milk supply have failed.

If you are expressing regularly for your pre-term baby you may have built up a stash of milk larger than your own baby needs. Some mothers feel that they would like to share this with other babies on the special care unit whose mothers cannot produce milk for their babies. In the unit you may find that you have shared stories and experiences with other families and feel that they have almost become your extended family. Don't forget that the units are full 52 weeks of the year and that when you and your precious baby have gone home to begin your new life as a family others will take your place.

There are Milk Banks run by the United Kingdom Milk Banking Association (UKAMB) across the UK and by HMBANA (Human Milk Banks of North America) in the USA. They collect and process breastmilk donated by mothers and distribute it to units to protect the smallest and most vulnerable babies. To be a breastmilk donor you will need to have some blood tests and complete a questionnaire to ensure that you are suitable. You will be asked about any medication that you are taking. Your milk will also be tested. In some cases you can take medication and breastfeed your own baby, but not donate. This is because milk supplied by UKAMB has to be suitable for all babies and it cannot be labelled in any way. If your own baby is exposed to a drug that you are taking through your breastmilk, the doctors caring for your baby will be aware of the potential effects. Babies receiving donor breastmilk need to have the purest possible milk, as no one would be able to differentiate between the effect of their own prematurity and the effect of a drug in however minuscule an amount in the milk. The most important effects are sedation, changes in blood pressure or changes in blood sugars.

It is known that the provision of donor milk, in the absence of the mother's own milk, reduces the risk of NEC by about 79%. This makes a significant difference to the number of babies who are seriously ill and may die. If you could provide this precious gift, a family of a premature baby would be very grateful.

Drugs you can take and still donate breastmilk:

- Paracetamol
- Asthma inhalers
- Progesterone-only pill
- Vitamins
- Folic acid
- Head lice treatment
- Indigestion remedies/antacids
- Loratadine (Clarityn) for hayfever
- Cetirizine (Zirtek) for hayfever if Clarityn does not work for you
- Nasal sprays to relieve symptoms of cold e.g. xylometazoline (Otrivine), Oxymetazoline (Vick Sinex)
- Nasal sprays and eye drops to relieve symptoms of hayfever e.g. Beconase, Opticrom
- Simple cough mixtures i.e. ones which don't cause drowsiness and don't contain decongestants e.g. glycerine honey and lemon, simple linctus
- Sore throat lozenge e.g. Strepsils, Lockets, Tunes
- Loperamide (Imodium) for diarrhoea

- Moisturisers to relieve symptoms of eczema e.g. E45, Diprobase
- Bulk-forming laxatives e.g. lactulose to relieve symptoms of constipation
- Levothyroxine
- Omeprazole

Drugs which are not suitable to take and donate breastmilk, but which you can take and breastfeed your own baby:

- Treatments for threadworm – avoid donating for 48 hours (Ovex, Vermox)
- Aspirin-containing products (Disprin, Beechams Powders, some combination painkillers) – avoid donating for 36 hours if taken accidentally (should not be taken during breastfeeding at all, but single doses are unlikely to cause problems for your own baby)
- Chlorpheniramine to relieve symptoms of allergy or hayfever (Piriton)
- Codeine
- Anti-hypertensive drugs
- Anti-depressants
- Antibiotics

If you are taking other medication please discuss with your local milk bank, which will normally consult me.

Informal milk donation

Some people donate their breastmilk informally or accept donated breastmilk from other mothers. In some cases mothers nurse each other's babies, as has happened throughout history. Wet-nursing is an ancient profession and has often been highly valued and respected, as well as well paid.

However, with informal milk donation – especially if you pay for it by volume – there is no monitoring of quality (the milk might be watered down), sterile collection or monitoring of drug-taking by the mother. Arrangements are entered into with a level of trust. If the donor is your friend and you know her well then you may feel able to accept her offer, depending on how much you need the milk.

I know of one mother who needed milk from dairy-free mothers for a severely intolerant baby with other physical conditions after her own milk supply had declined. It is very much an individual decision but should be made with as much information as possible from the donating mother.

UKAMB and HMBANA screen for bacterial contamination in the milk and sometimes fat content. They don't screen for medication but ask for full details and of course the mothers do not get paid for the donations. Research has shown that milk donated freely is of high quality as it comes from mothers who are highly motivated to help others.

There seems to be an increasing market for human breastmilk for adults. Some of it is used for therapeutic reasons, in cases of food intolerances and illness, such as cancer and inflammatory bowel disease, while some is consumed by athletes who think it will help performance. Others want it for dubious sexual reasons, so if you offer to sell your milk online please be aware that you may get some odd responses.

Donating your milk for a sick or pre-term baby whose mother is unable to breastfeed is a truly wonderful gift. If you have more milk than your baby needs and your freezer is already full please consider it.

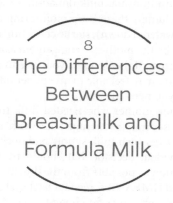

8
The Differences Between Breastmilk and Formula Milk

This message was recently posted on social media.

'Hi, a friend of mine recently told me that if she was prescribed medication, she would not breastfeed even if the medicine was considered safe, because she wouldn't want any "nasties" getting to her baby. Since this, I have done a bit of research and unless she opted for organic formula, most formulas (except soy and amino acid) are made from cows' milk, which comes from cows treated with artificial hormones and antibiotics. I thought I'd share this on here, as I know many of us are on medication and I often see posts from mums worrying about medication passing through their milk. Hope this might help put some minds at rest.'

The post made me think again about how we, as a society, perceive formula milk. The first things that came to mind were:

- Formula is the normal way to feed babies in the western/developed world
- It is used by most mothers before their babies are six months old
- It is recommended by healthcare professionals so it must be OK
- The adverts on TV say it is OK 'once you decide to move on from breastfeeding' and the babies always look OK
- I was formula fed and I'm OK
- Formula is scientifically made, it is always the same quality and it is tested
- It is easier for mum to get on with her life
- Dads don't feel so left out
- Formula feeding mothers get more sleep

I think I could carry on for several pages.

What about breastfeeding? Breastfeeding has been a major part of my life for the past 36 years. It is a passion. I make no apology for the fact that I don't understand why anyone would choose not to breastfeed. I know that things go wrong, that formula milk can be essential, that some women can't breastfeed even with all the support in the world and I don't want anyone to feel guilty about how they choose to feed their baby. This is truly not a book about blame. It is about support and the knowledge that sometimes I do have to tell mothers that they have to stop breastfeeding because they need to take a drug. For once in my life I am being honest about how I feel without putting my counselling hat on.

Unicef UK's Baby Friendly Initiative made a call to 'change the conversation' about breastfeeding in July 2016, saying:

> *'It is time to stop laying the blame for a major public health issue on individual women, and instead work*

together to build a supportive, enabling environment for women who want to breastfeed. It is time to change the conversation.'

Sue Ashmore, Baby Friendly UK Programme Director, blogged:

'Each time I write about breastfeeding I face a dilemma. On the one hand, there is more evidence than ever before that breastfeeding has long-lasting and profound benefits for both mother and baby. On the other hand, simply stating this fact causes pain and anger for the many families who tried really hard to breastfeed but were not able to. I really do understand that pain, because those people are also my own friends and family.

But does that pain and anger mean we ought to keep quiet about breastfeeding? Or should we do everything we can to remove those barriers which prevented women from successfully breastfeeding in order that more babies can be breastfed in future?'

Mothers need to be aware that all formula milks are the same regardless of cost or claims by the manufacturers. They are all composed of modified cows' milk (with the exception of some specialised milks necessary for infants with cows' milk protein intolerance). The manufacturers thus face a difficult task when developing and marketing their products; they have to produce a standardised, heavily-regulated product at an affordable price. Each company seeks to promote their brand by making it appear special and different to their competitors. Brand loyalty is encouraged.

There is no evidence that:

- Any brand of formula milk is superior to any other

- Switching from whey-to casein-dominant milk is necessary
- The introduction of follow-on milks is necessary
- The introduction of specially designed toddler milks is necessary

So what does make breastmilk different to formula milk? Breastmilk is a living fluid, which changes from hour to hour, day to day and month to month to meet the needs of the individual child. Breastmilk is more watery on a hot day or in a hot region to quench the thirst of the baby; it contains more fat in cold areas to keep the baby warm; it contains more protein if a baby is born pre-term to promote growth. Formula is always the same and this is sometimes thought to be a benefit – see my list above of how society perceives formula milk. However, in reality levels of some ingredients (such as added vitamins) may be higher or lower depending on how long the product has been on the shelf, and some ingredients are added, left out or changed depending on the price manufacturers must pay for them at any given time. (For more information see the work of First Steps Nutrition Trust.)

If a breastfeeding mother encounters an infection she will produce antibodies to that infection before the next feed in order to protect the baby. Amazingly, the baby's saliva changes if he/she meets an infection, inviting the mother to make antibodies to it and thus to protect her child.

Exclusive breastfeeding has been shown to reduce the risk of many infections:

- Less risk of gastroenteritis (Howie, 1990; Kramer, 2003; Quigley, 2007; Rebhan, 2009; Wilson, 1998)
- Fewer middle-ear infections (Aniansson, 1994; Duncan, 1993)

- Reduction in urinary tract infection (Marild, 2004; Pisacane, 1992)
- Fewer lower respiratory tract diseases (Bachrach, 2003; Ball, 1999; Howie, 1990)

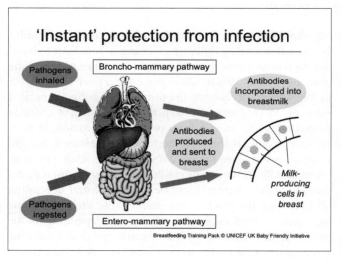

Entero-mammary and broncho-mammary pathway reproduced from UK BFI

This means that being formula-fed increases the risk of these infections. Interestingly the 2010 Infant Feeding Survey found that 83% of mothers cited 'best for the baby' as the reason for choosing to breastfeed, and 75% were able to name a benefit without prompting. Sadly only 17% were aware that breastfeeding also has important health benefits for the mother.

69% of women who were interviewed for the survey were aware that breastfeeding helps to build the baby's immunity.

Other health benefits frequently cited by mothers were that:

- breastfeeding reduces the likelihood of asthma, eczema and other allergies (25%)
- breastmilk is more nutritious and has more vitamins than infant formula (24%)
- the baby has less colic or wind and fewer stomach and digestive problems (13%)
- it helps to reduce the chance of childhood obesity (12%)

Reasons for choosing to breastfeed	Total %
Breastfeeding is best for health of baby	83
Breastfeeding is more convenient	22
Breastfeeding is better for mother's health	17
Closer bond between mother and baby	16
Breastfeeding is cheaper/free	15
Breastfed previous children	12
Breastfeeding is natural	11
Mother loses weight more easily	6
Influenced by health professionals	3
Enjoyed it, felt more comfortable/proud	2

Influenced by friends or relatives	2
History of allergies/illness in family	2
No particular reason	1
Other	8

Reasons given by mothers for choosing to breastfeed (McAndrew, 2012)

Of those mothers who stated that they planned to formula feed from birth, 56% were aware of the health benefits of breastfeeding and were able to name a benefit – but still chose to formula feed from birth. It is interesting to note the 10% who cited medical reasons for not breastfeeding – were these mothers told that they couldn't breastfeed because of medication or a medical condition? We don't know, as no further information is provided in the report.

Reasons for choosing to formula feed	Total %
Fed previous children with infant formula	21
Did not like the idea of breastfeeding	20
Convenient/due to mother's lifestyle	19
Other people can feed baby	17
Breastfed previous children and didn't get on with it/put off by others' experiences	11

Medical reasons for not breastfeeding	10
Would be embarrassed to breastfeed	10
Can see how much the baby has had	5
Had problems breastfeeding (unspecified)/not enough support[1]	4
No particular reason	4
Domestic reasons/coping with other children	3
Expecting to return to work/college soon	1
Feeding with infant formula is less tiring/is quicker	1

Reasons given by mothers for formula feeding from birth (McAndrew, 2012)

Breastmilk contains over 200 factors that we cannot replicate and thus are not found in formula milk. Our understanding of them and their importance for infant development is growing all the time. Below I discuss just a few.

Lactoferrin is a protein that binds to the iron present in breastmilk to help its absorption. Breastmilk has relatively low levels of iron, but the presence of lactoferrin allows it all to be absorbed (bacteria thrive in iron-rich environments). Formula milk has five to six times as much iron as breastmilk, but as it is in its free form (not bound to lactoferrin as there is none in formula), far less is available to the infant. Free iron supports the growth of bacteria and raises the risk of gastrointestinal infections, yet television ads often claim that follow-on formula milk provides more iron for the older baby. Mothers can't analyse their breastmilk, and they may doubt its quality thanks to misleading advertising.

Lactoferrin has several other functions, especially that it actively prevents bacterial growth. By binding to iron, it reduces levels available for bacterial growth. It also binds to receptor sites on the surfaces of bacterial cell membranes, causing the cells to break down and making replication impossible. Most importantly, it helps the cells lining the gut to stop foreign proteins passing through and causing damage. It isn't easily broken down in the gut, and stays intact to be found in the bowel motions of breastfed babies. Only 10% of lactoferrin is saturated with iron, leaving the remaining 90% free to exert its bactericidal activity.

Administration of supplementary iron to a breastfed infant interferes with this level of saturation, resulting in decreased bactericidal activity. However, iron supplements given to anaemic breastfeeding mothers do not interfere with the levels of lactoferrin in her breastmilk (Zavaleta, 2005). The concentration of lactoferrin is highest in colostrum and declines gradually over the following five months. The only time when exclusively breastfed babies need iron is if they are born very pre-term with inadequate stores of iron laid down during a pregnancy that was cut short.

Oligosaccharides act to coat the inside of the infant's gut, blocking the attachment of microbes and toxins. Any remaining pass on to coat the urinary tract, protecting it from infections too. Artificially-fed infants have fewer oligosaccharides in their bowel motions, and they are of a different composition to those found in breastfed babies. Although formula milk manufacturers claim to add oligosaccharides, the artificial ones have not been proven to have any benefit. Oligosaccharides may also be called prebiotics.

Lysozyme is an enzyme. It kills bacteria by causing a breakdown of their cell walls, so that effectively they explode. It also has anti-inflammatory activity. Levels increase during lactation, peaking at around six months. It has been suggested that this is to protect the gut during the introduction of weaning foods to the diet. It is found in large concentrations in the bowel motions of breastfed infants, but not those who are artificially-fed.

Epidermal growth factor seals the intestine, preventing the absorption of undigested protein and reducing the risk of allergy. It increases the production of lactase. It has been shown (Dvorak, 2003) that levels of epidermal growth factor are higher in many mothers who deliver extremely prematurely, compared to those who deliver prematurely, or at term, and that it may be involved in protecting the baby against NEC.

Secretory Immunoglobulin A (IgA) is believed to coat the gut, making it impermeable to pathogens and thereby protecting the baby. Concentrations are particularly high in colostrum. The tight junctions between the alveolar cells are wide open in the first few days after birth to allow free passage of the immunoglobulins to protect the baby. The cellular gaps gradually close over a few days to protect the baby from other substances, including drugs, getting through into milk. Other immunoglobulins in breastmilk are IgG, IgM, IgD and IgE.

Bifidus factor is a carbohydrate that promotes the growth of *Lactobacillus bifidus* which in turn inhibits the growth of harmful bacteria by encouraging an acidic environment, which is less conducive to pathogenic bacterial growth

Proteins in breastmilk, just as in formula, consist of two

types: whey and casein. Approximately 60% is whey, while 40% is casein. This balance of the proteins allows for quick and easy digestion. In formula there a greater percentage of casein, which is more difficult for the baby to digest, making the baby feel fuller for longer. Approximately 60–80% of all protein in human milk is whey protein. These proteins have infection-protection properties. So-called 'Hungry baby' formula milks have more casein than whey in the protein mix (80:20).

The fat component of human milk is highly variable and changes according to factors including the duration of feed, time since last feed, stage of lactation and the dietary habits of the mother (Agostoni et al, 1999). Fats are added to supply 50% of the energy in formula milks, and vegetable oils including rapeseed oil, coconut oil, sunflower oil and fish oils are used according to availability and cost.

Growth factors including Epidermal Growth Factor (EGF), Transdermal Growth Factor (TGF) and Inflammatory Growth Factor (IGF) have been identified in breastmilk. EGF is one of the major peptide growth factors present both in colostrum and human milk. Levels are highest in the first days after birth and then gradually decrease during the first two weeks. TGF-α is also present in human colostrum and milk, but at much lower concentrations than EGF. Neither is found in commercial infant formulas. Although the roles of these factors are not clearly understood, recent studies indicate the importance of these peptides in repair processes in injured intestinal mucosa and in prevention of NEC (Dvorak, 2003).

Leukocytes are white blood cells in breast milk, which engulf and destroy pathogenic bacteria. They are responsible for the longer time that expressed breastmilk can be stored.

Breast milk isn't sterile, but contains as many as 600 different species of various bacteria.

These are just a few of the ingredients which make

breastmilk unique to every mother and invaluable for the health of her baby. Knowing what we do, and with new research revealing further properties of breastmilk all the time, it's clear that we shouldn't be assuming that formula is fine if mothers need medication during lactation.

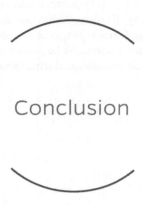

Conclusion

- Mothers' medication matters because women want to breastfeed (around 80% initiate breastfeeding at birth).
- Mothers' medication matters because babies deserve to be breastfed – their short and long-term health is better if they are breastfed.
- Mothers' medication matters for women's health too – women who breastfeed reduce their risk of disease, including breast cancer and osteoporosis.
- Mothers' medication matters because pregnancy and lactation are normal human states and mothers deserve to have their medical conditions treated and managed appropriately, just like everyone else.

Moderate increases in breastfeeding could save the NHS more than £40 million and result in tens of thousands of fewer hospital admissions and GP consultations (Renfrew, 2012).

It is in the interests of mothers, healthcare professionals and wider society that good, evidence-based information about drugs and medication is available and routinely accessed. I hope I have shown that there is evidence out there for the vast majority of drugs that should enable mothers to continue breastfeeding while obtaining the medical treatment they need. A change in our practice could have a huge impact on the health of future generations.

None of this is difficult. If we value breastmilk for its wonderful properties, practise evidence-based medicine and respect mothers, we could transform women's experiences of seeking treatment.

Mothers' medication matters! Maybe I'll have that engraved on my headstone.

'If breastfeeding did not already exist, someone who invented it today would deserve a dual Nobel Prize in medicine and economics'. Lancet, 2016

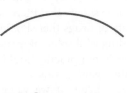

References

Agostoni, C., Marangoni, F., Bernardo, L., Lammardo, A.M., Galli, C. , Riva, E. Long-chain polyunsaturated fatty acids in human milk. Acta Paediatrica 1999; 88 (s430) : 68–71

Anderson, P.O., Pochop, S.L., Manoguerra, A.S. 'Adverse drug reactions in breastfed infants: less than imagined'. *Clin Pediatr* (Phila) 2003;42(4):325-40.

Aniansson, G., Alm, B., Andersson, B., Håkansson, A., Larsson, P., Nylén, O., Peterson, H., Rignér, P., Svanborg, M., and Sabharwal, H. 'A prospective cohort study on breast feeding and otitis media in Swedish infants'. *Pediatrics & Infectious Disease Journal* 1994;13: 183-188.

Aubrey-Jones, H.A., 'Evaluation of The Breastfeeding Network E-learning pack for GPs about Breastfeeding', 2012 University of Southampton Medical School final year undergraduate project.

Bachrach, V.R., Schwarz, E., and Bachrach, L.R. 'Breastfeeding and the risk of hospitalization for respiratory disease in infancy: a meta-analysis'. *Archives of Pediatric & Adolescent Medicine* 2003;157(3): 237-243.

Ball, T.M., and Wright, A.L. 'Health care costs of formula-feeding in the first year of life'. *Pediatrics* 1999;103: 870-876

Balon, A.J. 'Management of infantile colic'. *Am Fam Physician* 1997;55(1):235-42, 245-6.

Bandolier Infant colic update, 2004. www.medicine.ox.ac.uk/bandolier/booth/family/colicup.html

Bandolier Treatment for infant colic, 2000. www.medicine.ox.ac.uk/bandolier/band79/b79-4.html

Bartick, M., Reinhold, A. 'The Burden of Suboptimal Breastfeeding in the

United States: A Pediatric Cost Analysis' *Pediatrics* May 2010, 125(5) e1048-e1056.

Beilin, Y., Bodian, C.A., Weiser, J., et al. 'Effect of labour epidural analgesia with and without fentanyl on infant breast-feeding: A prospective, randomized, double-blind study'. *Anesthesiology* 2005;103(6):1211–1217.

Borra, C., Iacovou, M., Sevilla 'New Evidence on Breastfeeding and Postpartum Depression: The Importance of Understanding Women's Intentions'. *Maternal and Child Health Journal* 2015; 19(4): 897–907.

Boyd, C.A., Quigley, M.A., Brocklehurst, P. 'Donor breast milk versus infant formula for preterm infants: systematic review and meta-analysis'. *Archives of Disease in Childhood* 2007; 92:F169-F175.

Brimdyr, K., Cadwell, K., Widström, A., Svensson, K., Neumann, M., Hart, E.A., Harrington, S., Phillips, R. 'The Association Between Common Labour Drugs and Suckling When Skin-to-Skin During the First Hour After Birth'. *Birth* 2015; 42 (4): 319–328.

British National Formulary (BNF); Joint Formulary Committee. Online access www.evidence.nhs.uk/formulary/bnf/current

Chamberlain, G., Wraigt, A., Steer, P. (Eds). 'Pain and its relief in childbirth – the results of a national survey conducted by the National Birthday Trust 1993'. Edinburgh Churchill Livingstone: 49-68.

Cleugh, F., Langseth, A. 'Fifteen-minute consultation on the healthy child: breastfeeding'. *Arch Dis Child Educ Pract Ed* (epub 2016 http://ep.bmj.com/content/early/2016/07/28/archdischild-2016-311456.abstract).

Cover, D.L., Mueller, B.A. 'Ciprofloxacin penetration into human breast milk: a case report'. *DICP* 1990; 24(7-8):703-704.

Craig, W.R., Hanlon-Dearman, A., Sinclair, C., Taback, S., Moffatt, M. 'Metoclopramide, thickened feedings, and positioning for gastro-oesophageal reflux in children under two years'. *Cochrane Database Syst Rev.* 2004;(4):CD003502.

Dick-Read, G. *Childbirth without Fear: The Principles and Practice of Natural Childbirth.* Pinter & Martin, London, 2013.

Dixon, J.M. 'Treatment of breast infection'. *BMJ* 2011;342:d396

Duncan, B., Ey J., Holberg, C.J., Wright, A.L., Martinez, F.D., and Taussig, L.M. 'Exclusive breast feeding for at least 4 months protects against otitis media'. *Pediatrics* 1993;5:867-872.

Dvorak, B., Fituch, C.C., Williams, C.S., Hurst, N.M. and Schanler, R.J. 'Increased Epidermal Growth Factor Levels in Human Milk of Mothers with Extremely Premature Infants'. *Pediatric Research* 2003;54: 15–19.

Ebrahimi, N., Maltepe, C. and Einarson, A. 'Optimal management of nausea and vomiting of pregnancy' *Int. J. Womens Health* 2010; 2: 241–248. www.ncbi.nlm.nih.gov/pmc/articles/PMC2990891

EEC legislation 1989 (updated 2015). *Rules governing medicinal products in the European Community, Volume 2.* Notice to applicants for marketing authorisations for medicinal products for human use in the member states of the European Community. ec.europa.eu/health/documents/eudralex/

vol-2/index_en.htm

Einarson, A., Schachtschneider, A.K., Halil, R., Bollano, E. and Koren, G. 'SSRI'S and other antidepressant use during pregnancy and potential neonatal adverse effects: Impact of a public health advisory and subsequent reports in the news media'. *BMC Pregnancy Childbirth* 2005; 5: 11. www.ncbi.nlm.nih.gov/pmc/articles/PMC1156906/

European Monitoring Centre for Drugs and Drug Addiction. *Annual report on the state of the drugs problem in Europe*. www.emcdda.europa.eu/publications/annual-report/2012

European Monitoring Centre for Drugs and Drug Addiction. www.hscic.gov.uk/catalogue/PUB12994/drug-misu-eng-2013-rep.pdf

Fleiss, P.M. 'The effect of maternal medications on breast-feeding infants'. *J Hum Lact* 1992;8:7.

Gardner, D.K., Gabbe, S.G., Harter, C. 'Simultaneous concentrations of ciprofloxacin in breast milk and in serum in mother and breast-fed infant'. *Clin Pharm* 1992; 11(4):352-354.

Ghaffar, F., McCracken, G.H. 'Quinolones in Pediatrics'. In: Hooper, D.C., Rubinstein, E., (Eds) *Quinolone Antimicrobial Agents*. Washington, D.C., ASM Press, 2003: 343-354.

Giamarellou, H., Kolokythas, E., Petrikkos, G., Gazis, J., Aravantinos, D., Sfikakis, P. 'Pharmacokinetics of three newer quinolones in pregnant and lactating women'. *Am J Med* 1989; 87(5A):49S.

Global strategy on infant and young child feeding. http://apps.who.int/gb/archive/pdf_files/WHA55/ea5515.pdf?ua=12002

Gray, L. 'US study shows breastfeeding would save lives and money'. UNICEF Baby Friendly www.unicef.org.uk/BabyFriendly/News-and-Research/News/US-study-shows-breastfeeding-would-save-lives-and-money

Grayson, J. *Unlatched: The Evolution of Breastfeeding and the Making of a Controversy*, Harper Paperbacks, 2016.

Hale, T.W. and Rowe, H.E. *Medications and Mothers' Milk* (online access) 16th Ed, Hale Publishing, 2014.

Harmon, T., Burkhart, G., Applebaum, H. 'Perforated pseudomembranous colitis in the breast-fed infant'. *J Pediatr Surg* 1992; 27(6):744-746.

Harris, M. *Men, Love & Birth: The book about being present at birth your pregnant lover wants to read*. Pinter & Martin, London, 2015.

Heine, R.G. 'Gastroesophageal reflux disease, colic and constipation in infants with food allergy'. *Curr Opin Allergy Clin Immunol* 2006 Jun;6(3):220-5.

Hogg, M.I., Wiener, P.C., Rosen, M., Mapleson, W.W. 'Urinary excretion and metabolism of pethidine and norpethidine in the newborn'. *Br J Anaesth* 1977;49(9):891-9.

Howie, P.W., Forsyth, J.S., Ogston, S.A., Clark, A., and Florey, C.D. 'Protective effect of breastfeeding against infection'. *BMJ* 1990 300, 11-16, 52.

Hudak, M.L., Tan, R.C., 'The Committee on Drugs and The Committee on Fetus and Newborn. Neonatal drug withdrawal'. *Pediatrics* 2012;129(2):e540-60.

Hussainy, S.Y., Dermele, N. 'Knowledge, attitudes and practices of health professionals and women towards medication use in breastfeeding: A review'. *International Breastfeeding Journal* 2011;6:11.

Ito, S., Koren, G., Einarson, T.R. 'Maternal noncompliance with antibiotics during breastfeeding'. *Ann Pharmacother* 1993;27(1):40-2.

Jayawickrama, H.S., Amir, L.H., Pirotta, M.V. 'GPs' decision-making when prescribing medicines for breastfeeding women: Content analysis of a survey'. *BMC Res Notes* 2012 3(1): 82.

Jones, W. *The role of pharmacists in supporting breastfeeding mothers who require medication during lactation.* PhD thesis, University of Portsmouth, 2000.

Jones, W. 'Question from practice: Constipation after a caesarean section'. *The Pharmaceutical Journal* 2012; 288:715.

Kaguelidou, F., Turner, M.A., Choonara, I. et al. 'Ciprofloxacin use in neonates: A systematic review of the literature'. *Pediatr Infect Dis J.* 2011;30:e29-37.

Kanabar, D., Randhawa, M., Clayton, P. 'Improvement of symptoms in infant colic following reduction of lactose load with lactase'. *Journal of Human Nutrition and Dietetics* 2001;14: 359-363.

Koren, G., Moretti, Kapur, B. 'Can venlafaxine in breast milk attenuate the norepinephrine and serotonin reuptake neonatal withdrawal syndrome?' *JOGC* 2006 April; 28(4):299-302.

Koren G, Cairns J, Chitayat D, Gaedigk A, Leeder SJ. Pharmacogenetics of morphine poisoning in a breastfed neonate of a codeine-prescribed mother. *Lancet* 2006 Aug 19;368(9536):704.

Kramer, M.S., Guo, T., Platt, R.W., Sevkovskaya, Z., Dzikovich, I., Collet, J.P., Shapiro, S., Chalmers, B., Hodnett, E., Vanilovich, I., Mezen, I., Ducruet, T., Shishko, G., and Bogdanovich, N. 'Infant growth and health outcomes associated with 3 compared with 6 months of exclusive breastfeeding'. *Am J Clin Nutr* 2003; 78; 291-2959: e837-842.

LactMed A TOXNET DATABASE. Drugs and Lactation Database US Library of Medicine https://toxnet.nlm.nih.gov/cgi-bin/sis/htmlgen?LACTMED

Lee, A., Inch, S., Finnigan, D. *Therapeutics in Pregnancy and Lactation,* Radcliffe Medical Press, 2000.

Lida, H., Conrad, P., Adams, C. 'The effects of clinical aromatherapy for anxiety and depression in the high risk postpartum woman – a pilot study. Anxiety and depression markers compared to a control group'. *Complement in Ther Clin Pract* 2012;18(3):164-8.

Lucassen, P.L.B.J., Assendelft, W.J.J., Gubbels, J.W., van Eijk, J.T.M., van Geldrop, W.J., Knuistingh Neven, A. 'Effectiveness of treatments for infantile colic: systematic review'. *BMJ* 1998; 316: 1563-1569.

Ludman, S., Shah, N., Fox, A.T. 'Managing cow's milk allergy in children', *BMJ* 2013;347:f5424.

Lumbiganon, P., Pengsaa, K., Sookpranee, T. 'Ciprofloxacin in neonates and its possible adverse effect on the teeth'. *Pediatr Infect Dis J* 1991; 10(8):619-620.

Marild, S., Hansson, S., Jodal, U., Odén, A., and Svedberg, K. 'Protective effect of breastfeeding against urinary tract infection'. *Acta Paediatrica*, 2004; 93(2): 164-168.

Matheson, I., Kristensen, K., Lunde, P.K. 'Drug utilization in breast-feeding women. A survey in Oslo'. *Eur J Clin Pharmacol* 1990;38(5):453-9.

Mazzotta, P.L., Magee, L.A. 'A risk-benefit assessment of pharmacological and nonpharmacological treatments for nausea and vomiting of pregnancy'. Drugs 2000 ;59(4):781-800. As reported in Festin, M. 'Nausea and vomiting in early pregnancy'. *BMJ Clin Evid* 2009; 2009: 1405.

McAndrew, F., Thompson, J., Fellows, L., Large, A., Speed, M., Renfrew, M.J. *Infant Feeding Survey 2012.* digital.nhs.uk/catalogue/PUB08694/Infant-Feeding-Survey-2010-Consolidated-Report.pdf

McConnachie, A., Wilson, P., Thomson, H., Ross, S., Watson, R., Muirhead, P., Munley, A. 'Modelling consultation rates in infancy: influence of maternal and infant characteristics, feeding type and consultation history'. *Br J Gen Pract* 2004;54:598-603.

Metcalf, T.J., Irons, T.G., Sher, L.D., Young, P.C. 'Simethicone in the treatment of infant colic: a randomized, placebo-controlled, multicenter trial'. *Pediatrics* 1994; 94: 29–34.

MHRA Codeine: restricted use as analgesic in children and adolescents after European safety review 2015. www.gov.uk/drug-safety-update/codeine-restricted-use-as-analgesic-in-children-and-adolescents-after-european-safety-review

Morrison, C.E., Dutton, D., Howie, H., Gilmour, H. 'Pethidine compared with meptazinol during labour. A prospective randomised double-blind study in 1100 patients'. *Anaesthesia* 1987;42(1):7-14.

National Institute for Health and Care Excellence (NICE) 2006. *Postnatal care. Routine postnatal care of women and their babies. Clinical guideline 37.* www.nice.org.uk/guidance/cg37?unlid=101242622520166214475

National Institute for Health and Care Excellence (NICE) 2014. *Clinical Knowledge Summary Colic – infantile.* http://cks.nice.org.uk/colic-infantile

National Institute for Health and Clinical Excellence (NICE) 2011. *Food allergy in children and young people. Diagnosis and assessment of food allergy in children and young people in primary care and community settings.*

National Institute for Health and Clinical Excellence (NICE). *Inducing labour. Clinical Guidance* 70 www.nice.org.uk/guidance/CG70

National Institute for Health and Clinical Excellence (NICE) 2013. *Clinical Knowledge Summary Nausea and Vomiting in Pregnancy.* http://cks.nice.org.uk/nauseavomiting-in-pregnancy#!references/-322922

National Institute for Health and Clinical Excellence (NICE) 2015. *Gastro-oesophageal reflux disease: recognition, diagnosis and management in children and young people.* www.nice.org.uk/guidance/ng1/ifp/chapter/reflux-in-babies

National Institute for Health and Clinical Excellence (NICE) 2008. *Maternal and Child Nutrition, Improving the nutrition of pregnant and breastfeeding mothers and children in low-income households.* www.nice.org.uk/guidance/ph11

Nelson, S.P., Chen, E.H., Syniar, G.M., Christoffel, K.K. 'Prevalence of

Symptoms of Gastroesophageal Reflux During Infancy. A Pediatric Practice-Based Survey'. *Arch Pediatr Adolesc Med* 1997;151(6):569-572.

Palmer, B. 'Infant Dental decay – is it related to breastfeeding?' www.brianpalmerdds.com/caries.htm

Parker, A., Coleman, R.E., Grady, E., Royal, H.D., Siegel, B.A., Stanin, M.G., Sostman, H.D., Hilson, A.J.W. 'SNM Practice Guideline for Lung Scintigraphy 4.0' *J Nucl Med Technol* 2012;40(1): 57-65.

Pisacane, A., Graziano, L., and Zona, G. 'Breastfeeding and urinary tract infection'. *Journal of Pediatrics*, 1992;120:87-89.

Pole, M., Einarson, A., Pairaudeau, N., Einarson, T., Koren, G. 'Drug labelling and risk perceptions of teratogenicity: a survey of pregnant Canadian women and their health professionals.' *J Clin Pharmacol* 2000;40(6):573-7.

Quigley, M.A., Kelly, Y.J., and Sacker, A.S. 'Breastfeeding and hospitalization for diarrheal and respiratory infection in the United Kingdom Millennium Cohort Study'. *Pediatrics* 2007; 119: e837- e842.

Rajan, L. 'The impact of obstetric procedures and analgesia/anaesthesia during labour and delivery on breastfeeding'. *Midwifery* 1994;10 (2):87-103.

Rebhan, B., Kohlhuber, M., Schwegler, U., Fromme, H., Abou-Dakn, M., and Koletzko, B.V. 'Breastfeeding duration and exclusivity associated with infants' health and growth: Data from a prospective cohort study in Bavaria, Germany'. *Acta Paediatrica* 2009;98: 974-980.

Renfree, C. (Ed) 'Herbal Galactagogue Use for the Breastfeeding Mother'. *In Proceedings of ILCA Conference*, Scottsdale, AZ, USA, 2004.

Renfrew, M.J., Pokhrel, S., Quigley, M., McCormick, F., Fox-Rushby, J., Dodds, R., Duffy, S., Trueman, P., William, A. 'Preventing disease and saving resources: the potential contribution of increasing breastfeeding rates in the UK'. 2012 www.unicef.org.uk/Documents/Baby_Friendly/Research/Preventing_disease_saving_resources.pdf?epslanguage=en

Saha, M.R., Ryan, K., Amir, L. 'Postpartum women's use of medicines and breastfeeding practices: a systematic review'. *Int Breastfeeding Journal* 2015;10:28.

Sale, J.E.M., Gignac, M., Hawker, G. 'How "bad" does the pain have to be? A qualitative study examining adherence to pain medication in older adults with osteoarthritis'. *Arthritis Rheum* 2006;55: 272-278.

Salman, S., Sy, S.K., Ilett, K.F. et al. 'Population pharmacokinetic modeling of tramadol and its o-desmethyl metabolite in plasma and breast milk'. *Eur J Clin Pharmacol* 2011.

Salvatore, S., Vandenplas, Y. 'Gastroesophageal reflux and cow milk allergy: is there a link?' *Pediatrics* 2002 Nov;110(5):972-84.

Savilahti, E., Launiala, K., Kuitunen, P. 'Congenital lactase deficiency. A clinical study on 16 patients'. *Arch Dis Child* 1983;58:246-252.

Scott, J.A., Robertson, M., Fitzpatrick, J., Knight, C., Mulholland, S. 'Occurrence of lactational mastitis and medical management: A prospective cohort study in Glasgow'. *International Breastfeeding Journal* 2008; 3:21.

Shannon, M., Lacouture, P.G., Roa, J., Woolf, A. 'Cocaine exposure among children seen at a pediatric hospital'. *Pediatrics* 1989 Mar;83(3):337-42.

Sheikh, A., Tunstall, M.E. 'Comparative study of meptazinol and pethidine for the relief of pain in labour'. *Br J Obstet Gynaecol* 1986 Mar;93(3):264-9.

Sim, T.F., Hattingh, H.L., Sherriff, J., Tee, L.B. 'The use, perceived effectiveness and safety of herbal galactagogues during breastfeeding: a qualitative study'. *Int. J. Environ. Res. Public Health* 2015, 12: 11050-11071.

Sim, T.F., Hattingh, H.L., Sherriff, J., Tee, L.B. 'Perspectives and attitudes of breastfeeding women using herbal galactagogues during breastfeeding: a qualitative study'. *BMC Complement Altern Med* 2014 Jul 2;14:216.

Sim, T.F., Sherriff, J., Hattingh, H.L., Parsons, R., Tee, L.B. 'The use of herbal medicines during breastfeeding: a population-based survey in Western Australia'. *BMC Complement Altern Med* 2013;13:317.

Slowie, D. 'Doctors should help their patients to communicate better with them'. *BMJ* 1999;319:784.

The Academy of Breastfeeding Medicine Protocol Committee. *ABM Clinical Protocol #9: Use of galactagogues in initiating or augmenting the rate of maternal milk secretion* (first revision January 2011). *Breastfeed Med* 2011; 6;41–49.

Torney, Patrick (Harry), Oct 1992, M. Dent. Sc Thesis: *Prolonged, On-Demand Breastfeeding and Dental Decay - An Investigation*, Dublin, Ireland.

Units Health and Social Care report from the Personal Social Services Research 2013 www.pssru.ac.uk/project-pages/unit-costs/2013/

Vandenplas, Y., Brueton, M., Dupont, C., Hill, D., Isolauri, E., Koletzko, S., Oranje, A.P., and Staiano, A. 'Guidelines for the diagnosis and management of cow's milk protein allergy in infants'. *Arch Dis Child* 2007;92:902-908.

VanderVaart, et al. 'CYP2D6 polymorphisms and codeine analgesia in postpartum pain management: a pilot study'. *Ther Drug Monit* 2011; 33(4):425-432.

Venter, C. 'Cows' milk protein allergy and other food hypersensitivities in infants. *J Family Health* 2010. www.jfhc.co.uk/cows_milk_protein_allergy_and_other_food_hypersensitivities_in_infants_20679.aspx

Webb, J.A., Thomsen, H.S., Morcos, S.K., Members of Contrast Media Safety Committee of European Society of Urogenital Radiology (ESUR), 'The use of iodinated and gadolinium contrast media during pregnancy and lactation'. *Eur Radiol* 2005;15(6):1234-40.

Wessel, M.A., Cobb, J.C., Jackson, E.B., Harris, G.S., Detwiler, A.C. 'Paroxysmal fussing in infancy, sometimes called "colic"'. *Pediatrics* 1954; 14: 421-434.

Wilson, A.C., Forsyth, J.S., Greene, S.A., Irvine, L., Hau, C., and Howie, P.W. 'Relation of infant diet to childhood health: Seven year follow up of cohort of children in Dundee infant feeding study'. *BMJ* 1998;316(7124): 21–25.

Woolridge, M.W. and Fisher, C. 'Colic, "overfeeding", and symptoms of lactose malabsorption in the breast-fed baby: a possible artifact of feed management'. *Lancet* 1988; ii:382-384.

Zavaleta, N. Iron and Lactoferrin in milk of anaemic mothers given iron supplements. Nutrition Research 2005; 15(5):681-690.

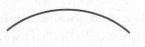

Resources

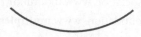

Breastfeeding helplines

National Breastfeeding Helpline: 0300 100 0212

Association of Breastfeeding Mothers: 0300 330 5453

The Breastfeeding Network (in English or Welsh): 0300 100 0210
    Bengali and Sylheti: 0300 456 2421
    Tamil, Telegu and Hindi: 0300 330 5469

La Leche League GB: 0845 120 2918

National Childbirth Trust: 0300 330 0770

Websites

Association of Breastfeeding Mothers **www.abm.me.uk**

Baby Milk Action **www.babymilkaction.org**

Best Beginnings **www.bestbeginnings.org.uk**

Bliss **www.bliss.org.uk**

Breastfeeding and Medication
    www.breastfeeding-and-medication.co.uk

The Family Planning Association **www.fpa.org.uk/home**

First Steps Nutrition Trust **www.firststepsnutrition.org**

GP Infant Feeding Network (GPIFN) **www.gpifn.org.uk**

Healthy Start **www.healthystart.nhs.uk**

Kathy Dettwyler **kathydettwyler.weebly.com**

Kathleen Kendall-Tackett **uppitysciencechick.com**

La Leche League **www.laleche.org.uk**

Maternity Action **www.maternityaction.org.uk**

Milk Banking Association **www.ukamb.org**

Multiple Births Foundation **www.multiplebirths.org.uk**

National Breastfeeding Helpline
  www.nationalbreastfeedinghelpline.org.uk

National Childbirth Trust **www.nct.org.uk**

NHS and breastfeeding
  www.nhs.uk/Conditions/pregnancy-and-baby

NHS Start for life **www.nhs.uk/start4life**

TAMBA **www.tamba.org.uk**

The Breastfeeding Network
  www.breastfeedingnetwork.org.uk

Tongue Tie Practitioners **www.tongue-tie.org.uk**

UNICEF Baby Friendly Initiative **www.babyfriendly.org.uk**

Index

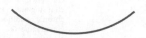

Why Mothers' Medication Matters

'baby blues' 58
Baby Friendly (UNICEF) 21, 147–8
Balon, A.J. 101
Bandolier 102, 104
beclometasone 67
beer 100
beta-blockers 40, 52
bifidus factor 155–6
biological norm, breastfeeding as 16
bipolar disorder 74–5
bisacodyl 68
blessed thistle 99
blood clots 40–4, 84
blood pressure 39–40, 52, 78
blood sugar levels (baby's)
        anti-hypertensives 39–40
        and beta-blockers 52–3
        and colostrum 53
        and fenugreek 100
        withdrawal symptoms 50
blood thinners 41
blood transfusions 39
Borra, C. 59
Botox 88
Boyd, C.A. 140
brand names versus generics 125
breast implants 88–9
breast pumps 130, 135
breast reduction surgery 88–9
Breastfeeding and Medication (Jones, 2013) 125
Breastfeeding Network 21, 126, 142
breastmilk *see also* colostrum; milk supply
        concerns about not enough 78–80, 98–100
        concerns about 'purity' of 15–18
        differences between breastmilk and formula 146–57
        donor milk 142–5
        factors not present in formula 153–7
        and gut health 16, 113, 154–6
        incidence of adverse events due to drugs in 54–5
        reasons for breastfeeding (mothers') 151–2
        syringe/ spoon feeding 37
        and tooth decay 85–6
Brimdyr, K. 34
British National Formulary (BNF) 20, 124
bromocriptine 44–6, 137
budesonide 67

cabergoline 44–5, 137
caesarean sections 34–5, 40, 68
calcipotriene 69
calcium 115
cancer 9–10
cannabis 82
carbamazepine 77
casein 115, 149, 156
cellulitis 93
central nervous system depressants 55
cephalosporins 122
Chamberlain, G. 35, 36
chamomile 99
chemotherapy 136
children, drugs prescribed for 67–8, 124
chlorpheniramine 144
choosing not to take medication 17, 18
chronic conditions 24–5, 54–77, 121
cinnarazine 66
ciprofloxacin 132–4
citalopram 71
clinical expert reports 19
clinical knowledge summaries 106
clinical trials 10, 13, 37, 102, 119
clobazam 77
clonazepam 77
clots (deep-vein thrombosis) 40–4
cocaine 81, 123, 135
codeine 62–3, 64, 66, 144
cognitive behavioural therapy (CBT) 58, 59, 71, 74
colic 101–6
Colief (lactase drops) 104–6
colonoscopy 75
colostrum
        beneficial factors in 154, 155, 156
        boosting baby's blood sugars 40, 53
        expression during pregnancy 25
        lactoferrin 154
        pregnancy whilst breastfeeding 32
        and syntometrine 39
        syringe/ spoon feeding 37
complementary and alternative medicines 40, 71–2, 99–100
conscious sedation 75, 87
constipation 35, 68, 109, 111
contraceptives 47–8, 136, 143
corticosteroids 69, 70
co-sleeping 81
cosmetic procedures 87–8
cough mixtures 143
cows' milk protein allergy/ intolerance (CMPA) 101, 108, 112–17

170

Index

Why Mothers' Medication Matters